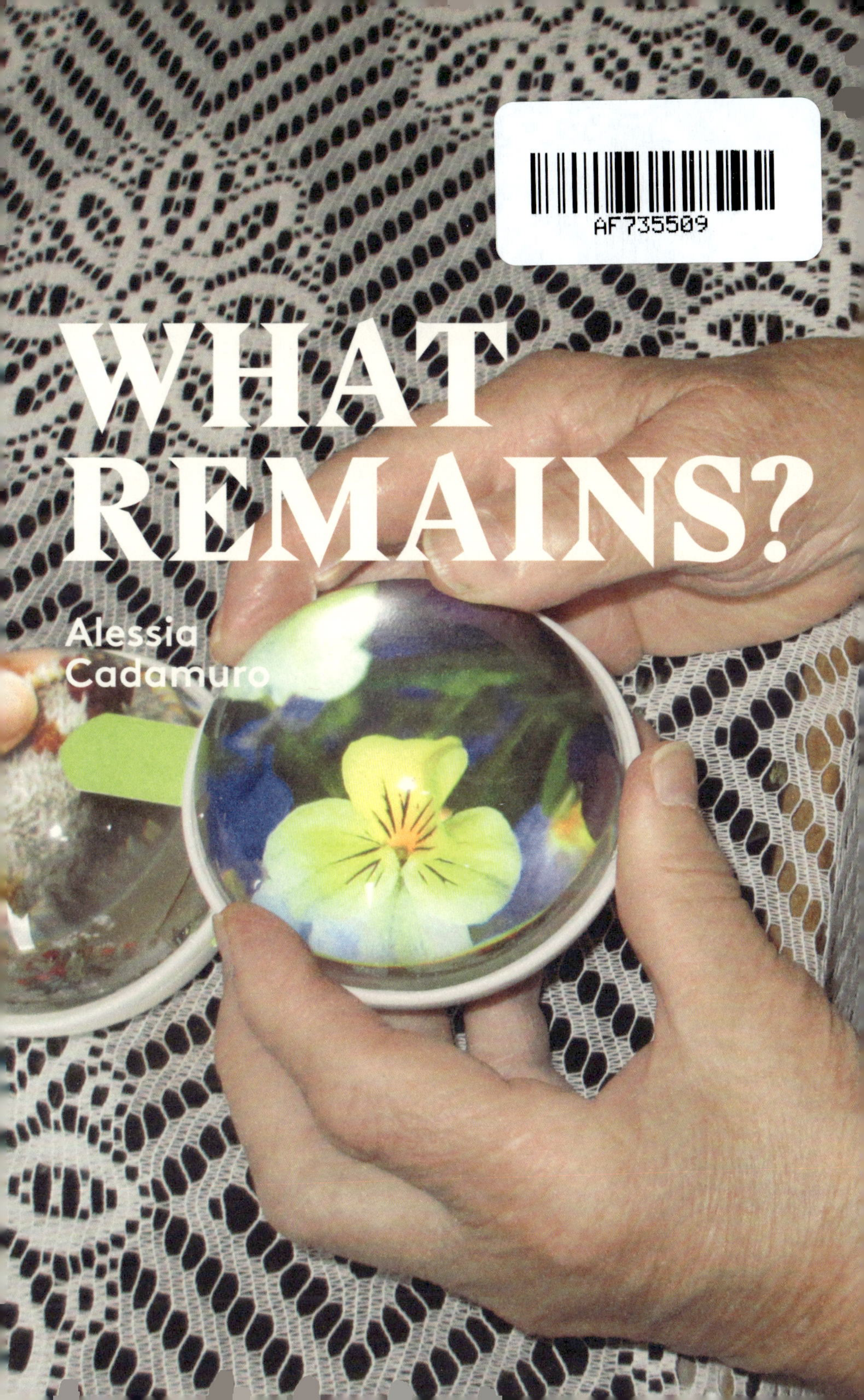

WHAT REMAINS?

Alessia Cadamuro

Contents

Designing for Dementia

Ré Dubhthaigh

In a world of increasingly older populations, the impact of Dementia on individuals, families and entire countries is only beginning to be understood. It is both a personal and societal challenge, altering relationships and changing the nature of care services. With predictions of 115 million people living with the condition, globally, by 2050, Dementia is forcing us to re-think old age and to develop new economic, social and cultural models.

Designers are taking on these societal challenges in a groundswell, working with others to develop new approaches to ageing, care and personal agency.

The UK Design Council's Living Well with Dementia challenge, The Helen Hamlym Centre, and the work of individual designers such as Alice Osborne (p. 41) represent a rich body of work; they see Dementia not as a technical or service delivery problem to be solved, but as a set of personal and professional relationships that need to be supported. These designers start with the people living with Dementia, building on the personal agency and needs of those most affected. Examples of such projects include Dementia Dog, a service that uses dogs to support the routines of Dementia sufferers. This programme was developed by a consortium including Alzheimer Scotland and the Glasgow School of Art as part of the Design Council's Living Well with Dementia challenge. Imagine: Dementia Dog Kaspa, who lives with Ken and Gynys; she helps reduce Ken's anxiety by supporting set routines in the day, such as getting out of bed or going to the shops.

Gregor Timlin and Nic Rysenbry's work at the Helen Hamyln Centre deals directly with the care home context. By exploring the care home environment the designers suggest a number of changes to support the cognitive, social and physical needs of residents, from new room layouts, to lighting, to tableware. Seemingly mundane redesigns of a cup or plate can vastly improve the experience of eating. By tackling the challenges of visual impairment and reduced dexterity, the designers help people retain agency over their lives.

Design projects that are driven by social innovation empower citizens by giving them the opportunity to co-design and co-produce their own solutions.

Ezio Manzini, founder and coordinator of DESIS, an international network of design for social innovation and sustainability, defines design for social innovation as a constellation of design initiatives geared to making social innovation more probable, effective, long-lasting and apt to spread (p. 53). He expands on this notion, by starting at the core: how design education institutions are the agents for such change.

Inspired by the idea of seeing the elderly as an asset for the whole of society, Virginia Tassinari set up the DESIS Cluster Project entitled *Ageing and Ingenuity* together with Yanki Lee and Sara Hylten-Cavalliuson. The DESIS cluster is an international group of projects of design institutions working on social innovation. Tassinari outlines the urgency to change our attitudes to senior citizens and to regard them as truly beneficial and essential members of society – assets, in fact (p. 47).

What Remains? fits within this body of work, building on the practices of designers in this space and adding new knowledge and expertise. In a similar vein to the projects outlined above, it has been co-developed with people who suffer from Dementia, moving beyond a traditional design approach of initial research followed by prototyping. Here, people are not defined as mere 'users' but active participants in the design process.

This involves deep engagement and points to new role for the designer as facilitator, translator and partner. It also emphasises qualities such as empathy and humility, a wider understanding of context and the ability to see design as a team sport rather than a solo endeavour.

Alessia Cadamuro, like her contemporaries, puts these news roles and qualities into action. It is the emphasis on impact that helps situate this work at the forefront of design for Dementia. Too often solutions can be overly focussed on technical fixes, but *What Remains?* concentrates on meeting real human needs and supporting personal interaction. Technology, indeed design, is an enabler rather than the goal.

What Remains? has already demonstrated impressive results, even within the limited scope of the prototype. Cadamuro's work with a mother and son has had a lasting impact on their relationship, helped uncover new insights to reduce anxiety in the care home, and can act as a memorial and repository for the family, after her death. Many design-led products and services for Dementia focus on early to mid stages of the illness, sign-posting to services and helping improve independence. This project expands on this existing work by showing the impact of design at later stages of Dementia. It has directly supported people with late-stage Dementia, encouraging a person to speak (meaningfully) for the first time in a number of years. In addition, it can identify meaningful stimuli, such as music, that resonate when other forms of communication are no longer possible.

Perhaps most importantly, *What Remains?* provides an example of how design can bridge the systemic and the intimate, linking larger scale challenges of service delivery with the personal interactions of close family members. In designing on these two scales, Cadamuro balances the needs of the system to gather actionable information with the desire of families to strengthen personal bonds.

By moving beyond bland personalisation and focussing on real people with real histories, *What Remains?* helps family and staff humanise care home services for the benefit of all concerned. For designers, and especially those working in sensitive areas such as Dementia, the ability to work in the space between the system and the individual is crucial, responding to and re-shaping the requirements of each player. Cadamuro's work provides a strong case for how design really can make a difference to both.

After co-creation, something must remain Introduction

Alessia Cadamuro

What remains when people's lives are affected at the late stages of Dementia? This particular disease is nowadays a delicate and important topic, because of the growing number of people facing Dementia – this year alone in the Netherlands an estimated 256,000 elderly people suffer from this disease, a reported 6,000 more than in 2012 [1] – and our need for ethical reflections and functional solutions as part of effective pastoral care.

The severest impact on patients' health at the hands of Alzheimer's disease (the most common form of Dementia), is that the sufferer is robbed of the ability to speak, move, remember or even eat. The difficulties in communication and understanding between elderly Alzheimer patients, carers and the elderly person's relatives, provokes in the patient a deep state of anxiety and aggression in every day life. Furthermore, Alzheimer patients regress together with their memory, and past events become their present reality. Detached from their present, their more recent memories, their abilities and their families, Dementia patients do not have the capacity to control their lives. The responsibilities fall back on their loved ones, care homes and on society at large. For this reason it is necessary to respect their dignity as individuals, by providing for their needs.

The *What Remains?* research was conducted within CRISP (Creative Industry Scientific Programme), which is a Dutch national research programme of more than 60 organisations, in which Design Academy Eindhoven collaborates with the Technical Universities of Delft, Eindhoven and Twente, VU and UvA in Amsterdam and over fifty design companies and service providers in the Netherlands spanning eight projects. G-motiv is one such project, its researchers and partner companies provided the context for *What Remains?*. G-motiv designs persuasive game products for service-oriented markets in social, physical and mental healthcare domains. Among its service partners are companies, which provide elderly care such as the care homes of Careyn. This is where I met Swanny, a patient affected by Dementia, and her son, Tonko, both of whom have helped bring *What Remains?* much further.

The close collaboration with the care facility, Careyn, and its manager, Marja Dijkwel, was important to provide the necessary backing for this design research.

Jurgen Claassen, clinical geriatrician of the Alzheimer centre at Radboud University explains in a Radio 1 programme on Dutch radio that there is a need for a new surge in research on Dementia: "Research on Dementia is often narrow: there has been a lot of research on therapies that turned out *not* to work. [...] More money has now been freed for research that takes a different approach. Many institutions are looking into the disease and are searching for new methodologies of research." [2]

From the very outset, the stakeholders in *What Remains?* saw the value of establishing human connections to fundamentally generate a sense of trust and mutual respect among the subjects of this research project. Many people decided to share their personal, and quite often painful stories that, once filtered by co-designing activities, became empowering knowledge that the elderly, their loved ones, and the carers could finally use as a proactive resource.

Empathy, calmness and friendliness are necessary to connect with people suffering from the later stages of Dementia, where the sufferer is pushed to an almost full detachment from reality, as if there were no longer a person inside the physical body.

However, something remains.

If autobiographical pictures are placed in their vicinity, even a person at an advanced stage of Dementia would start to feel emotional, react by smiling; in fact after several months or even a year of silence, a patient may even utter the name of the subject in a picture. This is what visual stimulations can generate; music and touch can also generate other significant reactions. Something remains and whatever it is, is not just confused and fragmented information; on the contrary: taste, character, preferences, feelings and sensitivity are fully intact.

An empathic approach in design could allow these patients a much deeper knowledge of relevant topics, such as those with an important social value. In such a way, design could become a medium for creating benefits in people's lives, but also in the life of bigger communities. Strategies, systems, services and products are the design medium; however, a collaboration of a multidisciplinary team is absolutely essential to gain full comprehension of the theme.

In conclusion, the same initial question continues to acquire importance: what remains after completing a design project? Due to the social importance and the urgency of this topic there is something that absolutely must remain after a co-created design project, such as this one, has been dedicated to Dementia patients, their family members and carers. The following pages analyse and present some of the possible answers.

References

[1] Alzheimer Nederland. 2013. *We(e)tenschap: hoeveel mensen met dementia zijn er?*: http://www.alzheimer-nederland.nl/actueel/onderzoek/2013/januari/hoeveel-mensen-met-dementie-zijn-er.aspx. Accessed 6 October 2013.

[2] Radio 1. 2013. *De toekomst van dementia neemt het aantal gevallen toe*: http://www.radio1.nl/items/86216-de-toekomst-van-dementie-neemt-het-aantal-gevallen-toe. Accessed 6 October 2013.

Not in the same present

based on interviews with Alessia Cadamuro
James M. Boekbinder

Imagine: from one second to the next, you suddenly find that your normal environment has vanished, along with everything and everyone you know and love. You're in an unfamiliar place, full of strangers. You panic and try to leave, but strangers hinder your escape, forcing you away from the door...

People with Dementia don't share the present with others. They often live in a past reality – except when they wake up suddenly in the nightmare of a place full of strangers, a place they're not allowed to leave. Loved ones are confronted with a person who no longer even remembers them, so they lose hope and stop trying to communicate. Carers are faced with the task of restoring peace of mind to people who are agitated, aggressive and disruptive, but who can't understand what is happening, nor communicate about it.

It was through observing the distress of residents when they awoke suddenly into the present – and would try to force their way out of it – that I was struck the idea to focus on memory as a basis to find new ways of helping carers calm and reassure residents in these terrible moments. Or even to prevent these dread moments from happening.

Over the course of a year, I worked with elderly people, their family members and occasionally a carer, to co-create a 'storytelling game' in which residents and their loved ones collected, shared and arranged images using physical photo-cards and a computer application. We investigated these images, which often revealed biographical information, which in turn helped carers better understand some of the causes of distress.

This resulted in new ways for carers to restore the peace of mind of residents in distress. It gave the residents' loved ones a way to build new relationships with them, even in cases where the person had lost all memory of their shared history. And most importantly – it gave the residents back some small, but highly significant, pieces of their own autobiographical self and a sense of the importance of that self to others.

The following three stories have been selected because they embody the project *What Remains?* in all its complexity and potential.

Meaningful Play
Co-creating with Dementia patients, their family members and carers

Alessia Cadamuro

What Remains? is a design research project that uses game elements, such as playful engagement and co-creation activities, to connect elderly patients suffering from late-stage Dementia, to their family members and carers.

This playful engagement with the users uses the psychology of play, which stimulates a high emotional involvement where the players – especially the patient's relatives and carers – take an active role in the game, which promotes positive results. This is due in part to the fact that Dementia patients convert their thoughts into images, which afterwards are translated into words and real contexts by their relatives and carers. As a consequence, carers and people who are in close contact with a patient take on roles similar to that of a detective, where each picture can be assigned a specific meaning to help the framing of different, personal, real life stories. Sometimes carers can count on the contribution of a patient who tries to describe the pictures, and is then able to recall specific memories. However, this does not often happen, due to the challenging health conditions of late-stage Dementia patients.

Getting familiar with the past of a person suffering from Dementia would not only allow for good personalised care, but would also help carers to prevent negative behaviour which is often provoked by the disease. In turn, this would protect the dignity of the patient and the relationship with their loved ones. Aside from personalising and dignifying care, this design-research project aims to re-frame care home systems by introducing the facilitation of the intake process with patients. A consequence of this is behavioural change and quality of life benefits for patients, which has a knock on effect for carers and relations alike. Co-designing with carers added fundamental information and knowledge to the design process, thanks to their experience, while at the same time it helped them gain a deeper understanding of what design could do in a care environment.

The collaboration and the support of all the subjects involved in this project were fundamental to create value. Carers, but also Dementia patients and their loved ones could finally feel empowered by their own discoveries. This generated creative and interesting opportunities for *What Remains?*. The thorough co-design-research process, consisting of interviews and building a relation of trust with patients, caregivers and relatives resulted in building an offline and online game.

Reaping the benefits of high emotional stakes within the psychology of play

The analogue game and its digital components

The first prototype comprises of two stages and two mixed-media tools, which both strictly depend on each other. The first stage involves a computer application whose features are shared between the patient's relatives and the care home. This computer application works as a mind map tool, which the relatives of the patients are asked to use for collecting and uploading pictures that can offer important life information about the patients. Pictures and information are divided into different categories, including family, jobs, holidays, memories, hobbies, pets, religion, favourite food, things they do/do not like to do, and other categories that may be extended by the relatives. The carers are also invited to collect pictures and information centred on objects that the patient frequently mentions or which seem to provoke restlessness during the daytime. All the information uploaded to the computer application is accessible by the relatives as well as the carers, and each patient has their own file.

The *What Remains?* application should initially be used during the intake phase of elderly people in a care home, providing the carers with a good understanding of each new patient. Immediately after intake, the app can be used to consult the personal information of the patient to quickly personalise the type of care. The interface of the application is also designed to continuously facilitate the update of pictures by carers and relatives of the patient, through new and more detailed information and discoveries. As a consequence, the application becomes an important tool to support the work of the carers, who can quickly memorise visual information about the patients.

The second phase only starts once the patient's relatives finish uploading the majority of the pictures and information related to the patient's life. The relatives and the carers make a selection of 40 to 50 pictures based on the scenario offered by the application, which allows the pictures to be selected one by one from the categories and printed in a circular shape. The pictures are then cut out and inserted into the game's twenty spheres, which become the triggering elements in the 'psychology of play' of the elderly patient, their relatives and carers. The shape and materials for the game's spheres were designed as a result of the multiple co-creation sessions, where abilities and deficits of the patients were tested to create a triggering, playful experience. For example, the game pieces increase the visibility of pictures that had been inserted, as the glass spherical shape magnified the pictures' size. We shall refer to these game pieces as picture spheres.

Starting a game session

Each game session starts by firstly setting up a very important part of the game structure: the creation of the right game atmosphere. During this phase it is very important for the patient to select a quiet spot in the care home where they can sit with the carers, with a cup of tea or coffee.

After the picture spheres are laid out on the table, the game can start its active phase, directly involving the patient's senses. The play experience starts when the patient's relatives or the caregivers ask simple questions related to the pictures the patient is looking at. The pictures serve as motivational game-elements to generate a storytelling path.

In our project experiments, most of the time the patient would start shifting about groups of pictures to create physical connections between them: often behind such actions are autobiographical memories that obtain a translation into new images in the mind of the patient. From the group of patients that collaborated on this project, it became clear that each connection carried a specific meaning and a real memory for each of them. However, while the combinations of pictures was sometimes a complete mystery to relatives and carers, they became at the same time the element that triggered them to investigate the 'hidden memories' of their charges.

Once the patient's relatives commence investigation, the difficulty lies in the seeming impossibility to create a verbal communication channel with their loved one. In fact, most of the time, Dementia patients are no longer able to speak or clearly explain themselves, generating countless obstacles for a clear understanding of what they are thinking and feeling. Now the patient's relatives can start to understand the stories behind the connected pictures through the help of family members and old family friends. Such an approach does not

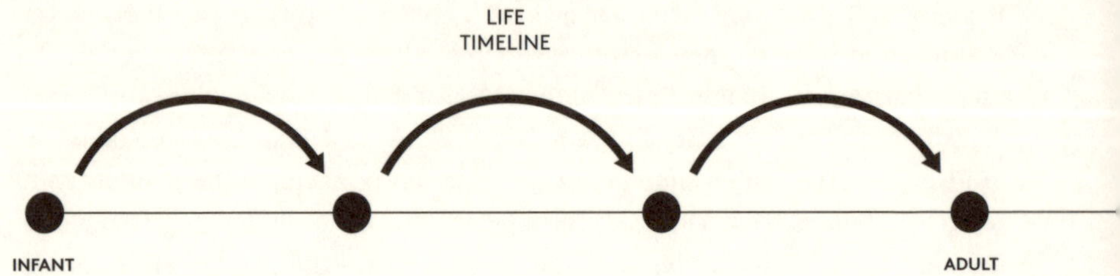
LIFE
TIMELINE
INFANT
ADULT

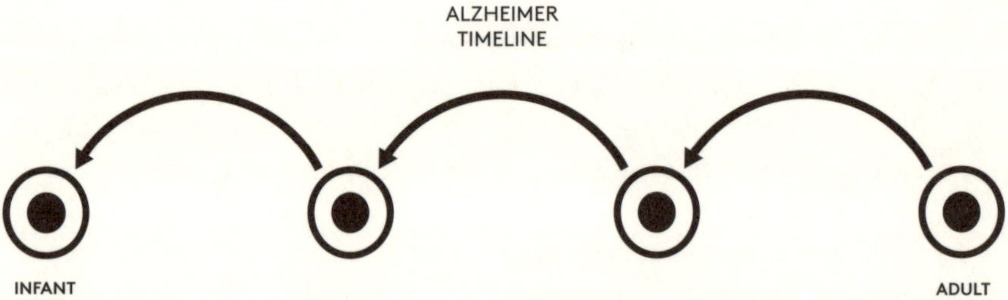
ALZHEIMER
TIMELINE
INFANT
ADULT

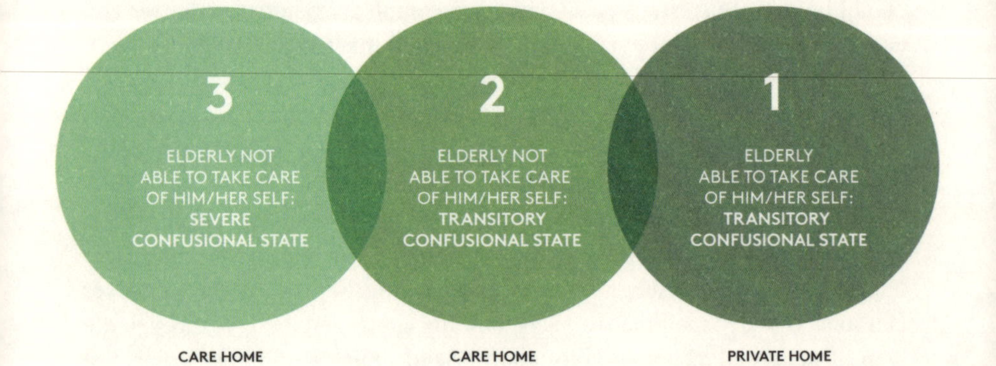
3
ELDERLY NOT ABLE TO TAKE CARE OF HIM/HER SELF: SEVERE CONFUSIONAL STATE
2
ELDERLY NOT ABLE TO TAKE CARE OF HIM/HER SELF: TRANSITORY CONFUSIONAL STATE
1
ELDERLY ABLE TO TAKE CARE OF HIM/HER SELF: TRANSITORY CONFUSIONAL STATE
CARE HOME
CARE HOME
PRIVATE HOME

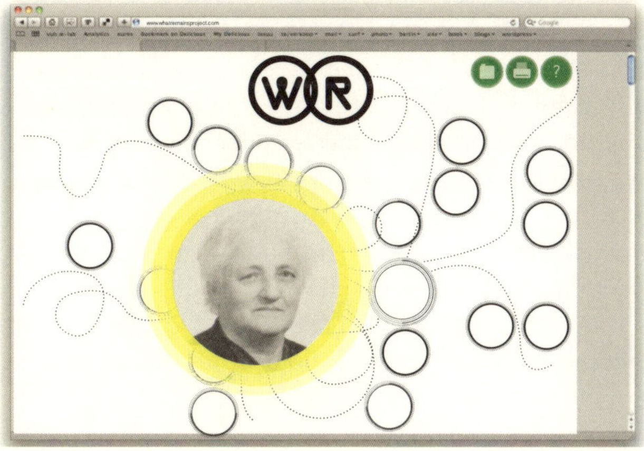

What Remains?
computer application, insertion of elderly with Dementia autobiographical images.

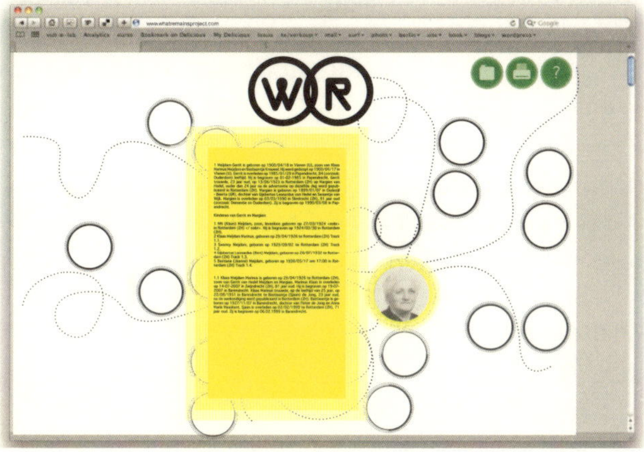

What Remains?
computer application, insertion of Dementia patients life stories.

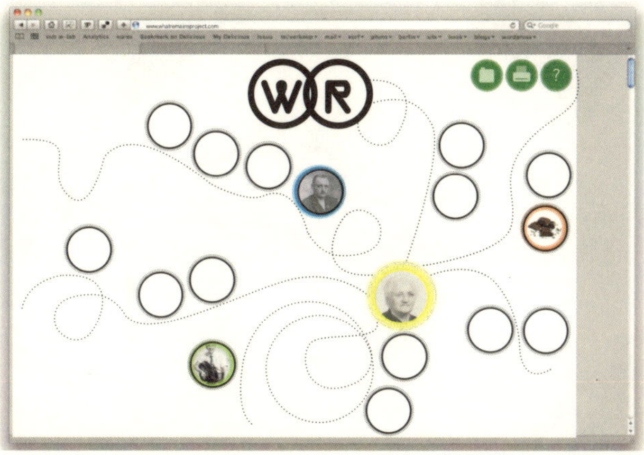

What Remains?
computer application, images insertion of different categories: subject, family, jobs, hobbies, pets, favorite food, things they did not like to do, things they do like, holidays, memories, other.

only empower the patient's relatives, but it makes them feel helpful, thereby strengthening the relationship between the family members and the patient in the care home. As such, the approach could be described as the perfect service... Each game session is documented by carers and relatives in a diary: a small booklet provided along with the *What Remains?* prototype. After each game session the carers can analyse the diary to personalise the care giving program for the patient and upload new information, and possibly pictures, on the application. Those recently added pictures would consequently become extra tools and, once printed out, they could be added to the game. They would then assist the generation of future sessions.

What Remains? guarantees a high level of control for the players, although the resulting stories are obviously unpredictable; this could potentially result in a situation that may get out of control. The game's merit lies in a continuous involvement of relatives and carers, aiming to better understand Dementia patients' thoughts via the impact of the stories, which are buried in their minds. *What Remains?* aims to re-frame part of the current care system for Dementia patients, looking for a personalised service able to improve the quality of life and communication in care homes. This approach is unique if we think about the current role of industries in the healthcare environment and specifically in Dementia care. *What Remains?* could be a bridge that connects Product Service Systems to the authentic intimacy of the users, enabling industries to support personal needs through their products.

What Remains? packaging.

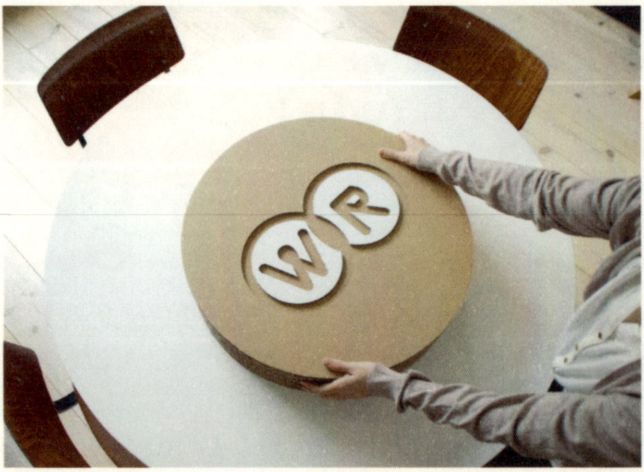

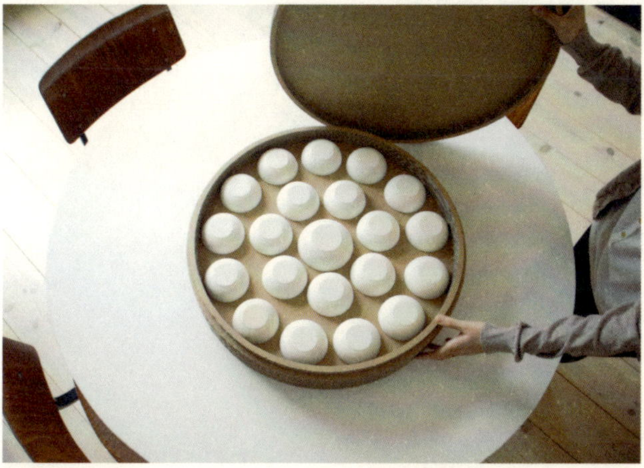

What Remains?
interior display.

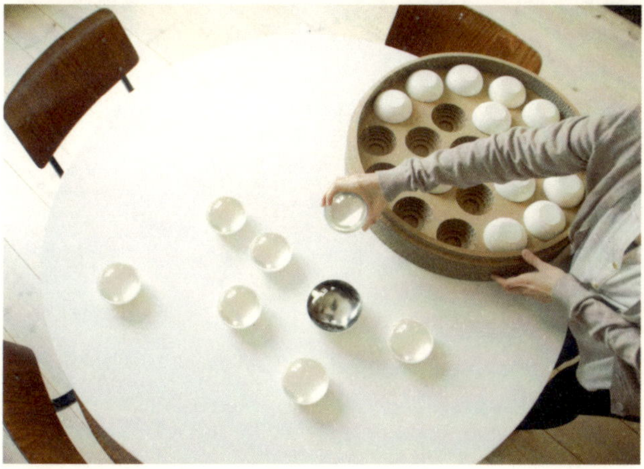

What Remains?
Picture spheres are displayed out of the box. The spheres are made from two materials: the top part is a semi-spherical magnifying lens and the lower part is plastic.

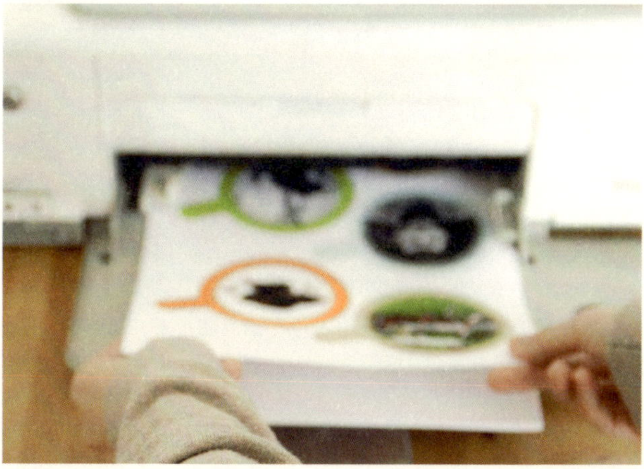

Personal pictures of Dementia patients previously uploaded in the *What Remains?* computer application are printed in the care home.

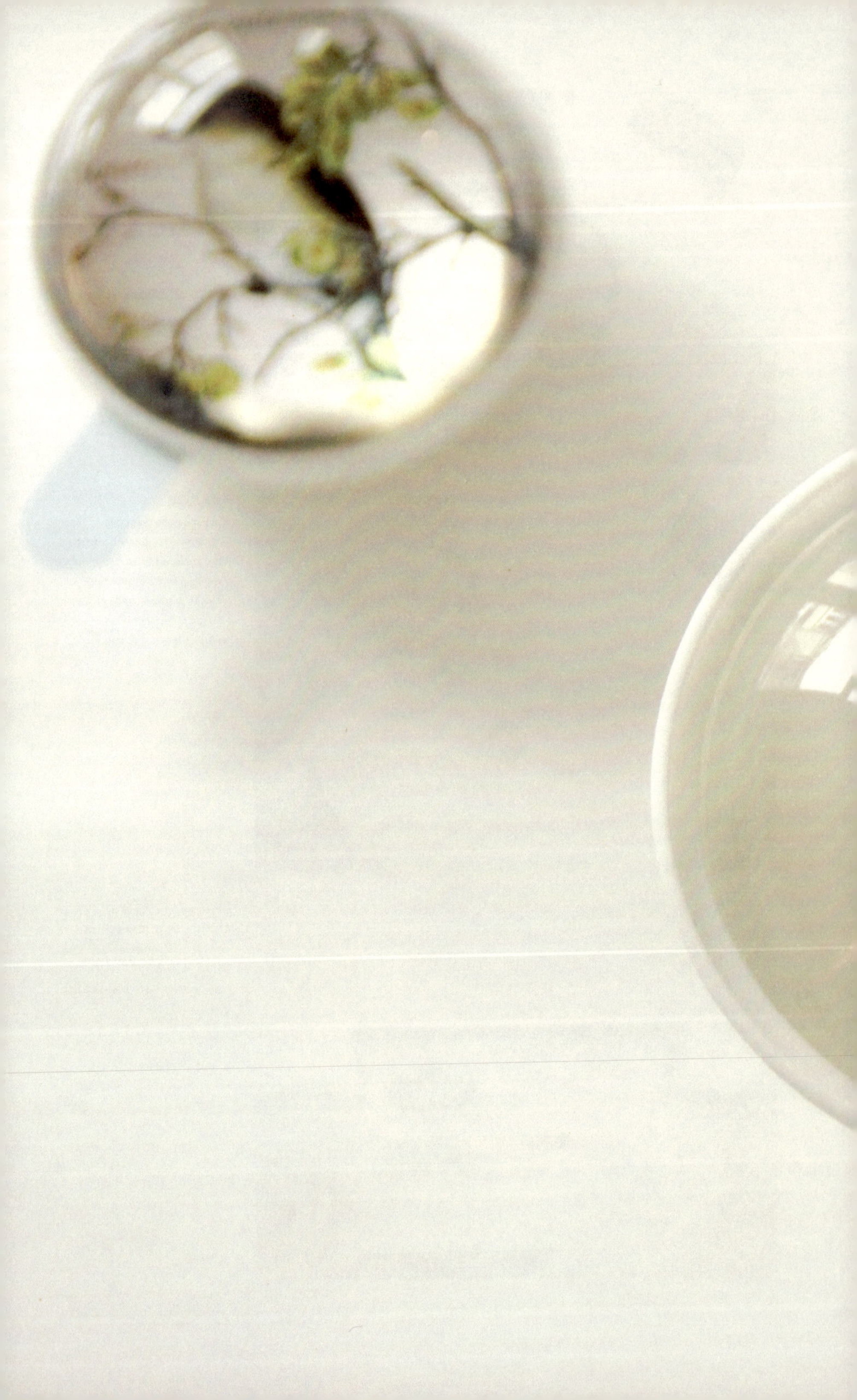

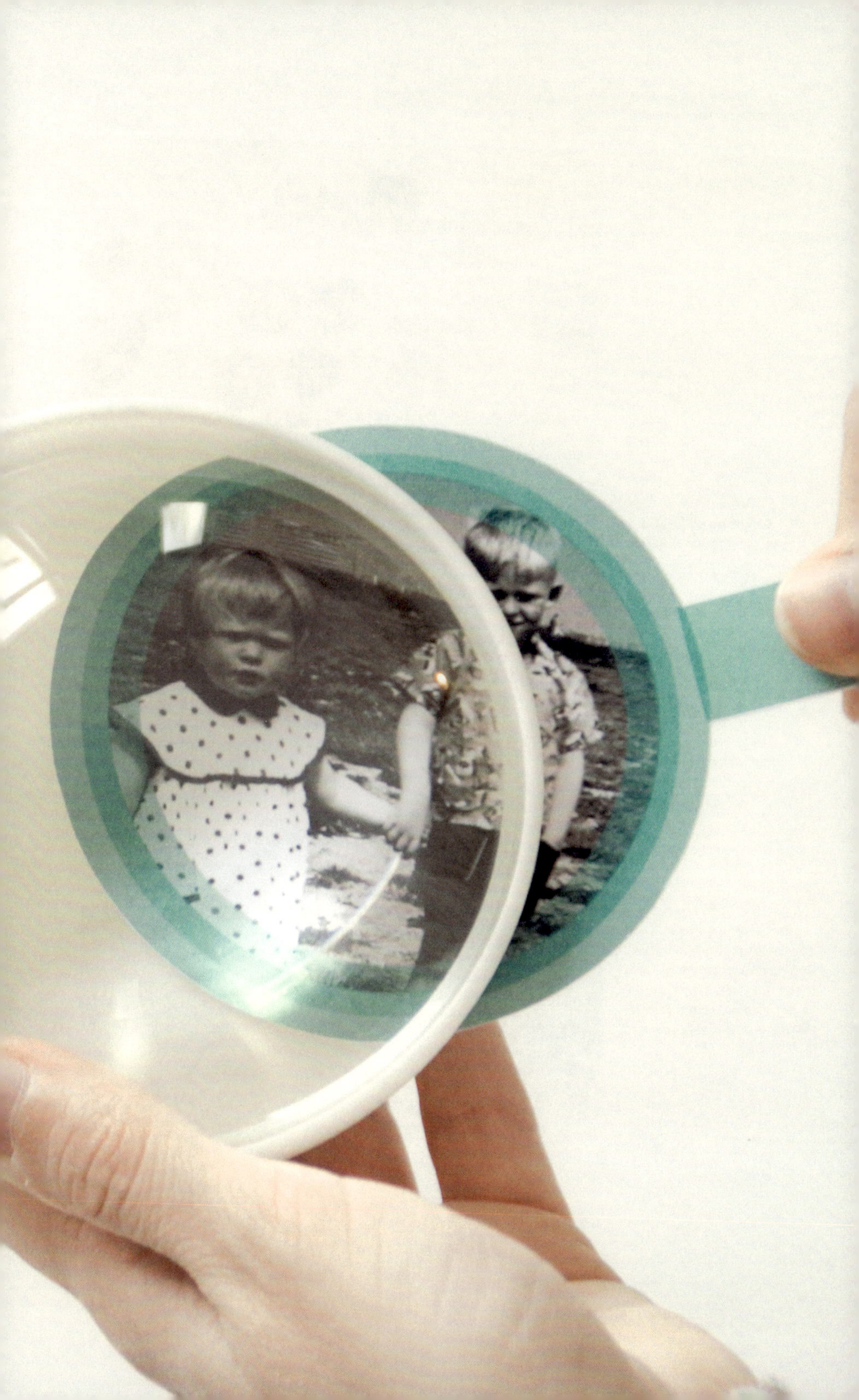

Personal pictures of Dementia patients are cut.

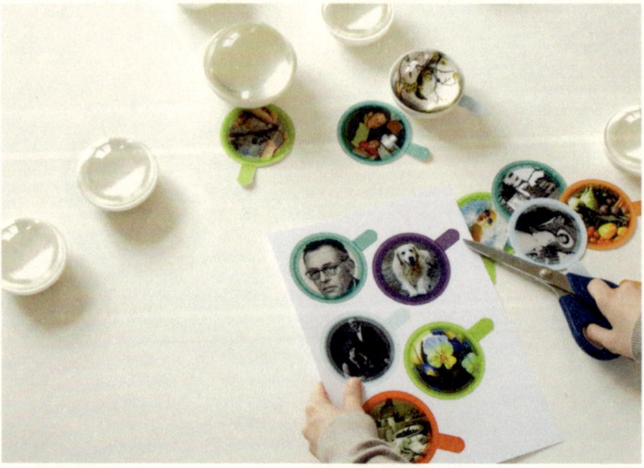

Personal pictures of Dementia patients are inserted into the spheres.

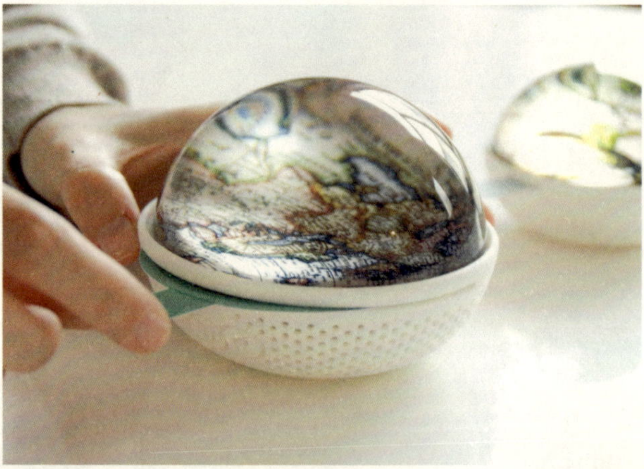

What Remains? storytelling game section with patients' personal pictures. Tender human contact and gentle caress are important for the patients during this activity.

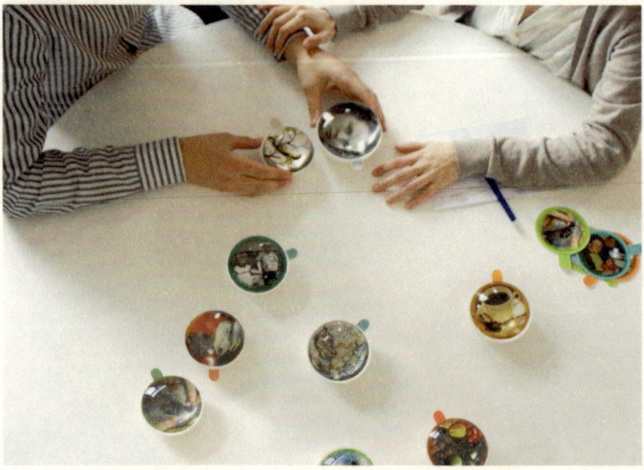

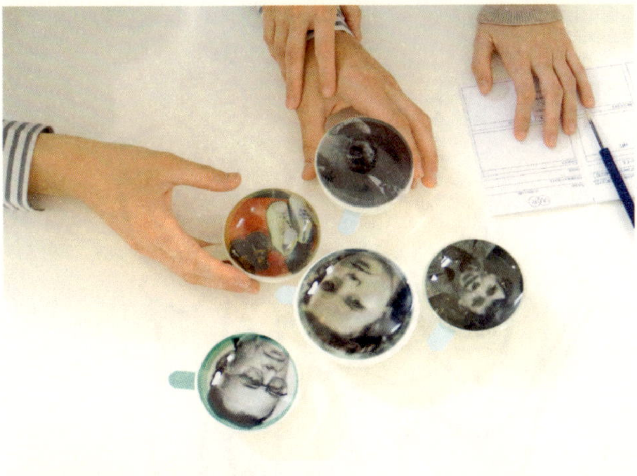

What Remains? storytelling game section with patients' personal pictures.

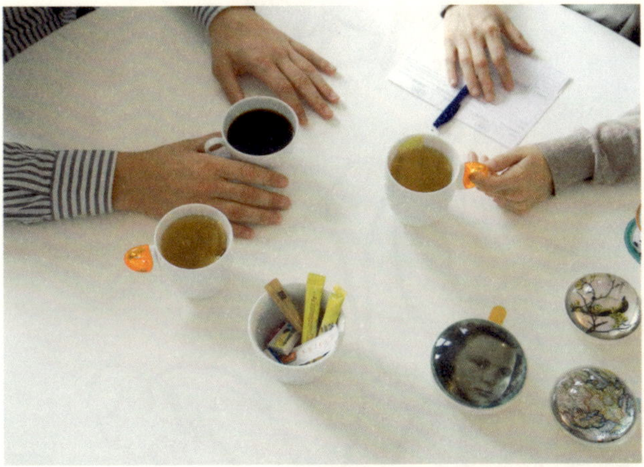

Tender human contact and gentle caress are important for the patients when playing the game. It is also important to start the storytelling in a comfortable and cosy atmosphere, for example with a cup of tea or coffee.

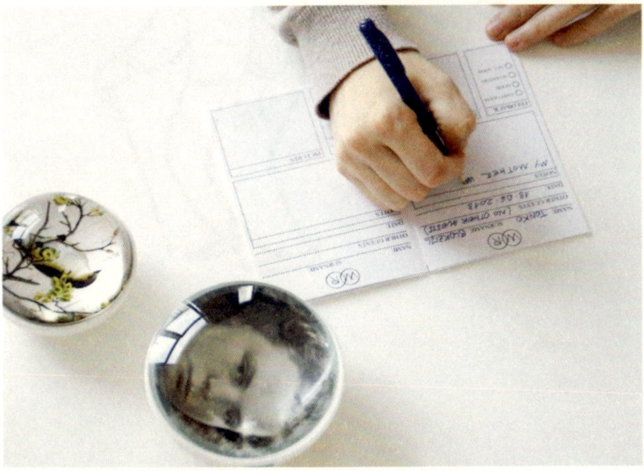

After each storytelling session carers or patient's family member write in *What Remains?* booklet about the image combinations created by Dementia patients, and any extra information relating to the story.

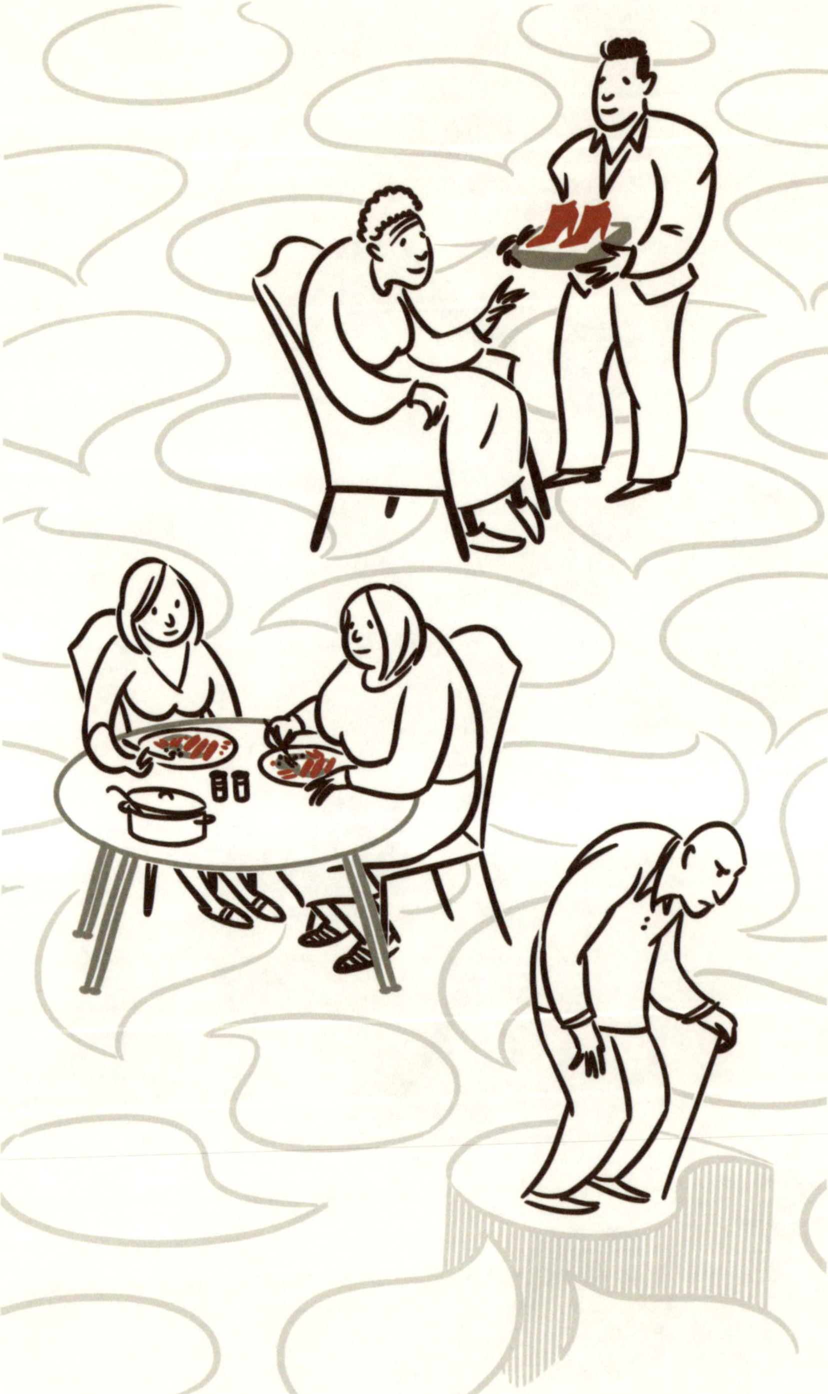

A second pair of shoes

Story 1 — Rita
James M. Boekbinder

Rita was often upset, especially in the morning, crying and demanding a second pair of shoes she claimed were stolen. Like all residents, she had one pair of shoes. We added a picture of shoes to the application, to try and find out more. In the course of several sessions, we noticed she put together this picture of shoes with a picture of her father. Her son investigated this, and found out from her sister that when they were girls, their father always bought them two pairs of shoes, one for everyday use, and one for special occasions and church. The son bought a pair of elegant dress shoes and the caregivers placed them next to her other shoes, beside her bed. From that moment, she stopped complaining about the shoes.

It was then that I understood the direction the project had to take. Perhaps she was re-living the time when she was between ten and fifteen years old – for her, that period in her life was the present. I realised that the information carers had about the residents was actually quite limited, and that if they could gain a deeper understanding of their memories, they might succeed in helping them feel more secure. To think - seemingly small things which held no great meaning for others could be of great help to these residents.

This simple, board-game-like activity, in which the resident made combinations of images on round cards, helped Rita communicate something which she couldn't put into words.

This began a positive, upward spiral in her relations with carers and family. The more they collected, investigated and discussed images, the more they found out. Her loved ones now had a way to be actively involved with her instead of only helplessly bearing witness to the disintegration of the person they had known. Rita was able to 'tell' some of the stories bottled up in her mind, previously unable to get out. Carers were able to save these stories in little books, which gave them topics to communicate with her about – themes for chatting, as it were, which engaged and reassured her. They discovered other ways to improve daily routines, including the way food was prepared.

Learning from real life experiences Interview with the son of a Dementia patient

Alessia Cadamuro

"I always had a great relationship with my mother, because she was easy to talk to and she was a very joyful person. When she started to show the first symptoms of Dementia it became difficult for me and my family to communicate with her and little by little she became a different person. With the progress of the disease, my relationship with my mother became more painful and difficult to manage. She was completely detached from the present and did not recognise me and my sister anymore." In this interview, Tonko Blokzijl describes the relationship with his mother, Swanny Meijdam-Blokzijl, who was affected by Alzheimer's disease. Tonko was one of the first family members who participated in *What Remains?* and who, together with his mother, enabled further development of this project.

Swanny lived in Hellevoetsluis, a Careyn care home; however, all the residents, their relatives and carers call this centre 'Polaris'. The care home is divided into six separate apartments, which accommodate six elderly residents with Dementia, each assisted by carers. Every patient shares the space with other elderly residents who have not only different types of Dementia, but are also at different stages of their diseases. The look of the apartments is warm and cosy and the furniture is neat, to make the residents feel comfortable and as though they might be living in their own homes. Sometimes the social dynamics are complex because six strangers are forced to live together and this can generate emotions and reactions such as competition, jealousy and antipathy. Despite this, the groups have the appearance of a family, and people become attached to each other quickly. This is where Swanny shared an apartment with five other women. She started her experience at Polaris when she began to manifest the first significant symptoms of Dementia, such as being unable to recognise her family, nor speak fluently, or take care of herself.

Tonko understood that his mother was progressively losing her memories and that the sole way to connect with her was by talking about the past. Quite often when he asked his mother to repeat or remember information about recent events, Swanny started to feel restless because she could not recall any new information. In the collaboration in *What Remains?* a patient's life-related pictures are important tools to stimulate communication with patients with Dementia. Tonko provided many different pictures from his mother's life, since he saw it as an excellent way for him to get to know her better. He also felt that the act of searching for images that could rebuild his mother's life story was a practical manner in which he could be more useful and involved in her life at the care home.

It was surprising for both of us to discover that existing pictures about Swanny's life could reveal important hidden memories and generate, as a direct consequence, peaceful as well as funny conversations with her. The discovery of hidden memories was also an unexpected, very important result for the project, while Tonko was very motivated to understand the meaning behind them. Seen from Swanny's perspective, it was only partially possible to explain the meaning of the photos, and most of the time it was quite hard to understand the complete story behind them. The difficulties in communication caused by the disease can often be an obstacle for the relatives of elderly people with Dementia, as well as for the carers. Together with Tonko, during and after several co-design sessions, we understood that his mother was using different pictures to translate her thoughts: it was the first time in several years that Tonko could understand what Swanny was thinking about. This triggered Tonko and motivated him to keep helping his mother to give voice to her hidden thoughts, and at the same time he gained a better understanding of her difficult behaviour, plus strategies to prevent it.

Tonko used all the information that his mother was able to communicate and started to look for information in many different directions such as consulting old family photo albums and talking with different family members. Thanks to his curiosity and ability to involve different family members, he was able to understand the meaning of connections between photos that Swanny made and shared with us. As a consequence of this activity Swanny really enjoyed looking at the pictures together with her son, because at those times she received a lot of attention and was able to feel important and loved once again. Her regular facial expression was rather serious, with a lost look in her eyes; but when she was with her son, using and looking at the pictures in *What Remains?* her expression was always different; she would smile and was clearly positively involved in the activity. Her motivation in communicating was growing to the point that she even started to joke about her past, remembering events and memories in a more active way.

By talking with Tonko it became clear that it was beneficial for him to collect pictures about his mother's life because this activity could re-generate the connection between the two of them. "Opening a new channel of communication with a person suffering from Dementia is a very important thing for the patient's relatives and carers. It is also very important to make use of an activity such as *What Remains?* because it can be very beneficial in the care home environment, where the relationships between the elderly and their loved ones are very difficult and painful. For me it was extremely beneficial especially because I had the opportunity to get closer to my mother again, and spend many beautiful afternoons with her looking at the pictures, talking and laughing. I still have all the images that I collected during the *What Remains?* sessions in my computer, and when I look at them I realise that they are connected to really nice memories and positive feelings. I hope that many other elderly people with the same disease, and their relations, might experience the same beneficial results through *What Remains?*. "

Deep understanding through interdisciplinary collaboration Interview with a Dementia care manager

Alessia Cadamuro

After several interviews with Marja Dijkwel, manager at Careyn care home based in the Netherlands, it was clear that memories play a very important role in the life of patients living in such facilities. Mrs Dijkwel described her experience of how elderly patients with Dementia spend most of their life inside their own memories, completely disconnected from the present and everything around them. The sharp contrast between patients' concepts of the real world and the recalled, fragmented memories often generates negative emotions in their minds, which provoke feelings of anxiety, fear and aggressiveness. From several observations at Careyn it was clear that such negative emotions can deeply influence the behaviour of Alzheimer's disease (AD) patients and that, for this reason, carers and relatives have difficulty finding a suitable communication channel with them.

Mrs Dijkwel employs the use of metaphors to describe how the human brain works when it is affected by Dementia: "You can compare our brain with many boxes that fit one inside the other, where the first box that we place inside will be also the last one to go out and vice versa. In this way it is easy to understand how our first memories will be the last to finally leave our brain." Autobiographical memories therefore become fundamental during the three different stages of Dementia. Past memories, for example, are extremely detailed in Dementia patients' mind; however, basics such as the capability to speak are often lost, decreasing a patient's fluency in communication. Mrs Dijkwel also outlined the world of a person suffering from Dementia as a fragmented world, where memories and emotions are trapped in their mind. Those memories and emotions are mostly disconnected, creating a lost feeling in the patient.

Concerning the importance of memories, the care home proposes places and activities that are related to the past. Some of them have what is called a 'memories room', a room containing old objects that reference the past; sometimes they encourage keeping a 'book of life', a blank notebook in which carers and patients can stick photos belonging to their past life; in some cases a personal photo album is used. Activities such as the 'memories room' or the 'book of life' are mostly intended as entertainment activities for elderly patients with Dementia. Mrs Dijkwel: "entertainment moments and activities are very important in a care home environment, to offer a patient a pleasant time. Memories could take on an important role if they were to be used to trigger the abilities and communication skills of the patients. With this understanding *What Remains?* could play an important role in care homes, since it stimulates elderly Dementia sufferers to communicate using their personal memories and it helps them to translate their inner world to family members and carers. A knock on effect for patients can also be to experience a positive change of behaviour and improvement in the quality of the relationship with their loved ones and carers. These outcomes are very important, especially when we look at the behavioural problems that patients with Dementia often face."

Mrs Dijkwel describes the relationship between Dementia patients and their loved ones as something similar to a long goodbye journey that generates painful emotions and a variety of relational complexities. For instance, for carers it is difficult to communicate to AD patients when they are restless. Often patients do not understand where they are and they try to escape, while screaming and crying. Sometimes they attempt to run out through doors or even windows, in their mind desiring to go home to see their parents. These moments of agitation for many patients occur due to a phenomenon called 'mirroring effect', whereby a patient literally mirrors the behaviour of somebody close who is attracting his attention. In those difficult moments a big role is played by carers.

Mrs Dijkwel introduced the job of carer as complex work that only trained personnel could do, which is of crucial importance to properly support stressful moments in a patient's life. Their role is positioned between patients and their families and they have a central position to understanding both parties.

All the subjects involved in this research project were fundamental in creating value through the co-design activities. This research methodology was a new experience for Mrs Dijkwel. In this case the introduction of co-designing activities into care home environments has certainly increased the understanding of the new role that designers can play to generate a better healthcare environment. Thanks to the understanding and support from the staff at Careyn it was possible to initiate an intense collaboration with elderly patients with Dementia, their relatives and carers.

Fear of falling

Story 2 — Paul
James M. Boekbinder

He expressed a fear of falling, and saw the carpeted floor as a chasm. He often talked about his past work as a farmer and carpenter. Was his fear of the floor related to memory? His own experience? Sharing images wasn't a good option – he was quick to become aggressive and our objective was to reduce distress, not increase it. We did succeed in understanding that the floor's colour provoked this fear. He seemed to think he would die if he fell.

His relatives' inquiries produced many stories, about his work and the traumatic death of a sister who drowned after falling into a canal. But it was unclear whether there was any connection between these incidents, or his former work, and his fear of falling. It could have been a product of his own brain – Paul had Vascular Dementia, which disrupted his balance.

The interaction with Paul taught us something about the limits of this approach when faced with the sheer complexity of a faltering brain. We didn't succeed in shedding more light on Paul's fear of falling and his distress. Hours of talking with his brother, wife and son had produced relatively little, and nothing like the flourishing new activity we'd seen with Rita.

However, carers paid special attention when choosing a material and colour for the floor of his dwelling. And being the centre of attention of his family – how important it made him feel, the affirmation of him as an individual – made a real difference in his quality of life.

In almost all the residents we worked with, we saw improvements in their state of mind. We learned to conduct the sessions in a private room instead of the common room, so that residents would feel more like the sole focus of attention.

A persuasive Product Service System to communicate between worlds

Valentijn Visch

G-motiv designs persuasive game products for service-oriented markets in the social, physical and mental healthcare domain. G-Motiv aims to show that persuasive game design can be effectively applied to respond to societal healthcare demands, one of which is aged care. Among G-Motiv's service partners are companies that provide aged care, such as Careyn in Brielle. This project attempts to investigate how persuasive game-based products might enhance existing care services. It should be stated that we do not develop complete Product Service Systems (PSS); we *add* a product to an existing service, leading to a result-oriented PSS [1]. The result (in this instance, care) is provided to the client and when the project finishes, it becomes possession of the company (Careyn) and is not to be further launched onto the market.

The care provided by Careyn is specialised to serve aged sufferers of Dementia among which Alzheimer Disease (AD) is the most frequently occurring one. A symptom of AD is the impairment of verbal communication abilities of the patient [4] making it difficult for the care provider to (a) *understand* the behaviour of the patient (e.g. why a patient is searching for her shoes constantly), (b) to *recognise* the care demands of the patient (e.g. when does a patient want care and when do they not), and (c) to *provide* the care to the patient (e.g. take a patient to the park). Summarised, the care-providing service is impaired by communication from patient to care provider, and vice versa. The user research within *What Remains?* showed that this communication problem is especially prevalent during the first months of the care-giving process. It takes about six months for the care providers to learn, by trial and error, how to understand the patient, recognise her care demands, and how to provide appropriate care. *What Remains?* aims to shorten this 'intake' period by facilitating the communication between patient and care provider during the intake process, through shared personal information about the patients' personal history (work, family, preferences, etc.).

The G-Motiv project focuses on the application of game-elements to motivate, persuade and help users towards a desired behaviour (i.e. for the context of *What Remains?* this relates to enhancing patient information for the care provider, during intake). In order to understand the design for such a game-mediated behavioural change, we developed the Persuasive Game Design model. This shows how gamification design motivates users to experience a game world so as to obtain 'behavioural transfer effects' in the real world [6] (see Figure 1). The user experience occupies a central position along the axis of a game world experience and a real world experience. Gamification design motivates the user to shift along this axis towards a game world experience by seducing her with motivating game elements such as fantasy or competition. In the specific context of *What Remains?*, however, the AD suffering patient may already have lost a grasp of the real world: patients in mild to moderate stages of AD have typically lost their ability to recognise their position in the world with regard to time and space [3]. Non-patients can easily discern the distinction between game and real worlds just as they can discriminate fiction from non-fiction [5]. Generally speaking, the enjoyment and freedom experienced in a game world may even be explained by its distinction from the real world: you might enjoy a game world because it is an escape from the humdrum of daily life or you might enjoy the fact that your actions and empathic relationships have less serious and long-term consequences in a fictional world than in the real world (such as shooting an opponent). In the case of the AD patient, however, this distinction between both worlds is less clear cut. They might not notice the difference between fantasy and real life or between game world experience and real world experience. As a consequence, the communication design of *What Remains?* should match the real world of the care provider to the game world of the patient.

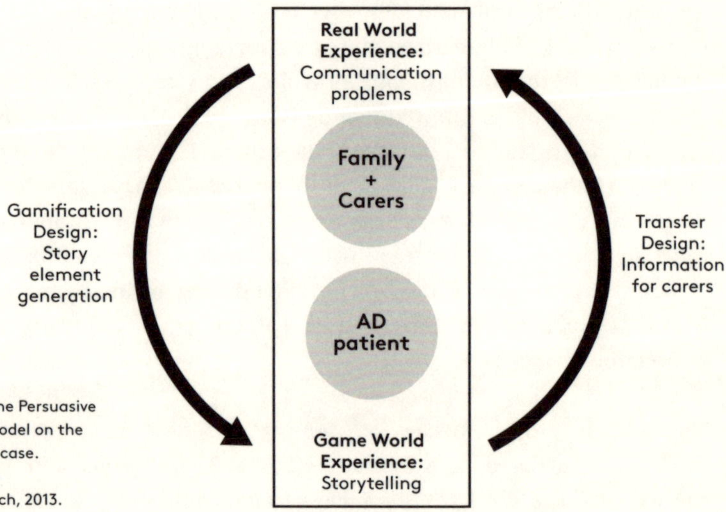

Figure 1:
Application of the Persuasive Game Design model on the *What Remains?* case.
– reprinted from Cadamuro & Visch, 2013.

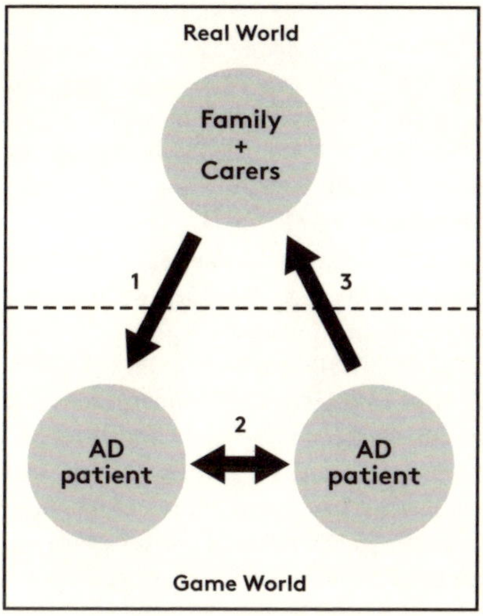

Figure 2:
Interaction processes
in *What Remains?*.

What is interesting about *What Remains?* are the sequenced interaction phases of users and product. In the first phase, family members and care providers upload personal pictures of the patient into the product. These pictures are collected from diverse media (photo albums, the internet) and are digitally uploaded to the *What Remains?* programme (based on Monobanda's 'Mindset' programme) - see arrow 1 in Figure 2. In the second phase, the pictures are printed onto circular pieces of cardboard which are inserted into transparent half-spheres and presented as objects - game pieces as it were - to the patients. Interestingly, the spheres modify the original flat, and difficult to grasp, pictures into graspable objects that show the pictures in a transformed and magically life-like manner - reminiscent of the nostalgic snow globe. The gamification of *What Remains?* thus consists of story elements that can be motivational for the user for the following four reasons: (a) the original picture content is related to the patient's life and may evoke re-living of specific memories, (b) the collection of pictures begs for connecting narratives, (c) the picture as object invites grasping, and (d) the pictorial transformation by the spheres may match the AD suffering patients' perceptual world experience. The motivational objects might lead to the behaviour found during the *What Remains?* research of patients interacting (grasping and grouping) with the object (arrow 2) and to tell the related connecting stories to the care provider and family member (arrow 3). Finally, this storytelling is transferred into valuable real world information for the family member (as remembrance) and for the carer (to understand, recognise and provide), as a personal, tailored care service.

References:

[1] Baines, T., Lightfoot, H., Evans, S., Neely, A., Greenough, R., Peppard, J., Roy, R., Shahab, E., Braganza, A., Tiwari, A., Alcock, J., Angus, J., Bastl, M., Cousens, A., Irving, P., Johnson, M., Kingston, J., Lickett, H., Martinex, V., Michele, P., Tranfield, D., Walton, I., & Wilson, H. (2007). State-of-the-art in product-service systems – review article. *Proceedings of the Inst. Of Mech. Engineers, Part B: J. of Eng. Manufacture, 221,* 1543-1552

[2] Cadamura, A., & Visch, V. 'What Remains?': A Persuasive Storytelling Game to facilitate intake of Alzheimer's Disease suffering patients in care homes. *GamesforHealth conference*, (Amsterdam, The Netherlands, 2013). In press.

[3] De Vriendt, P., Gorus, E., Bautmans, I., & Mets, T. (2012). Conversion of the Mini-Mental State Examination to the International Classification of Functioning, Disability and Health terminology and scoring system. *Gerontology, 58*, 112-9.

[4] Egan, M., Berube, D., Racine, G., Leonard, C., Rochon, E.: Methods to enhance verbal communication between individuals with Alzheimer's disease and their formal and informal care givers: a systematic review. *International Journal of Alzheimer's Disease*, doi:10.4061/2010/906818

[5] Visch, V., & Tan, E. (2009). Categorizing moving objects into film genres: The effect of animacy attribution, emotional response, and the deviation from non-fiction. *Cognition, 110(2)*, 265-272.

[6] Visch, V., Vegt, N., Anderiesen, H., vanderKooij, K. Persuasive Game Design: A model and its definitions. *CHI conference* publication, (Paris, France, 2013), http://gamification-research.org/chi2013/papers/

Fond of cooking

Story 3 — Ellen
James M. Boekbinder

Ellen was extremely passive. She barely responded to the people around her and no longer recognised her daughter. While initially hesitant about the project, her daughter uploaded a number of pictures and we did a session with her. A few of the images caused quite a response - Ellen opened her eyes wide, and became more animated, especially at the pictures showing food. Ellen had been quite fond of good cooking.

Ellen's daughter was surprised by her mother's response to these images of food and cooking, and also of dancing. We tried some music, and again, Ellen responded strongly to it. Her daughter realised that Ellen's love of food was still there. She decided to cook once a week for Ellen and the other six residents of the unit.

In Ellen's case, her daughter came to terms with the limitations Dementia imposed, and the session helped her create a new role for herself, in which she could positively influence her mother's life.

In conclusion...

Communicating with people with severe Dementia is extremely difficult.[(2)] I am convinced that the insights produced by our 'storytelling game' can play a critical role in providing truly personalised care. This becomes more important as late-stage Dementia sets in, and the channel of communication narrows. Personalised care means having more exact knowledge of what a person likes, needs, or doesn't... Residents, their loved ones and carers together can turn insights into interventions that greatly improve the residents' lives.

1. All names have been changed for reasons of confidentiality.
   Any resemblance to real persons is purely coincidental.
2. 'Severe' here refers to stage 2 and 3 Dementia.

Now is probably a good time

Alice Osborne

Intuitively I feel a resistance around sharing my experience of being a 'designer as change agent'. Because to tell the truth, it is really tough: I keep asking myself, "why do I bother?" Surely my life would be better/easier/freer if I made use of my pure design skills, and went to work every day 9 to 5 delivering posters to sell the next best thing. There is some weird and intrinsic part of my body – I don't think it is in my brain, but I am not entirely sure where I might locate this part of me. Perhaps it's my heart, or my gut that keeps me from the 9-5-next-best-thing job. It reminds me that I'm a natural innovator, I love seeing what's going on in the world, and dreaming and imagining how things can be better than they are.

In order to get from where we are, and move towards this vision of designer as change agent, there are a lot of tricky, difficult schemes to fill in. This part of me (the anti-9-5-er) also never lets me forget that I am one of those people who thrive on innovation, which means I generally work with people going against the grain. But you see, this is necessary to allow for new ideas or ways of thinking. For better or worse, I positively flourish in conditions that are tricky, and as much as my sub-conscious brain occasionally reminds me and says "Alice, this is your choice, get back to posters", I say, "No. Let's keep going and keep trying this slow road, in the hope it leads somewhere towards that vision."

Imagining the designer as change agent

The vision is centred around joined-up thinking, better integration of health and social care, and the creation of human-centred services as opposed to providers just 'providing'. I'd like to see a more collaborative approach to collectively working across all barriers in order to improve the way things work – systemically. I imagine the removal of blame within the health and social care system. Space for trying things out and being allowed to fail, the unleashing of creativity within individuals in an organisation and the reconnection of workers to their passion and drive. It also gives individuals within organisations the power to try, to be given permission to have a go at something new. I imagine care homes connected to their communities, having access to activities to help them prosper, and share resources, best practice and expertise across providers, as well as working towards having the capacity to answer people's needs based on quality, and not simply the ticking-off of tasks.

The journey is rocky and not easily defined but still I would rather travel it, waking up everyday, wondering what my imagined world would be like. I might be contributing, if even just a tiny bit. I'm working towards a bigger dream. (This stimulates the un-defined body part that likes tricky situations).

A designer from the beginning until the very end

My background is in graphic design but I have worked across health and social care, ageing, and end-of-life for the past six years. My passion is to work on projects that are forward thinking in their approach to help society live well, age, support independence, co-dependence, sharing and openness to the way we prepare for and face the end of our lives. Currently I am a design consultant for London Circle CIC, the design lead at My Home Life, creative director at Spots of Time and on the advisory board for Care Opinion. Previously, I was a designer at Thinkpublic with a range of clients including Carebase, the Department of Health, the NHS, the Alzheimer's Society, the Calouste Gulbenkian Foundation, U3A, Age UK, Mind and Timebank.

Designing for our futures

We are currently at breaking point in ageing. Never before has there been so much need to focus on it. The global population is booming, we are living longer and our health and social care landscape is changing. We are ill prepared for our future. Care home managers need to be good business thinkers, as well as carers. As care becomes more expensive, more emphasis is put on self-funding. As resources become more limited, and expectations become conversely greater, our aged care strategy is sitting precariously on a conveyor belt, headed toward unprecedented outcomes.

Sadly, health and social care is not quite as 'sexy' as other sectors demanding designers' skills, such as advertising or fast cars, or the latest Armani pyjamas. You see, I think that given the brain designers have, and its creative streak, we can apply its use to so many applications, not just fancy clothes, or cars or posters. What about a care home, a ward in a hospital, an estate? Right now some of my friends are designing alternative learning environments through community-making and production (makerversity.org), designing new opportunities in the area of early childhood care. (http://www.designcouncil.org.uk/our-work/challenges/health/the-knee-high-design-challenge/). They are setting up social enterprises like thegoodgym (http://www.goodgym.org/) to reduce social isolation as we age, and helping the sharing of food within communities (http://www.casseroleclub.com/).

The designer advantage

We must focus our strengths and our weaknesses in terms of what we can bring, and what we need help with, and need to get really good at talking about them. We should focus our attention as designers on how we can contribute our brain power, our way of being curious, being fearless about asking the bigger questions, our ability to visualise things and how we can facilitate and mediate discussions by directing people, and transforming passions from words into things. They might be products or services or websites - it doesn't matter, because it's the process of design-thinking and innovation that is the valuable part. A lot of my work is about trying to embed that mindset in the attitudes of local leaders.

Because we do things as we go, we are not afraid of failing, and we need to try things out to see what works, rather than solely researching it. Therefore, we can experiment fast, fail quicker and learn faster than in other projects, where lots of money can go into a small amount of rigorous research. We need to focus our efforts. Not everyone will be in the market for some Armani pyjamas, but it's a fact that we will all age, lose the people we love, need help to get dressed, lose teeth. We might develop Dementia, or cancer; we may need a care home; we will inevitably become frailer and lonelier, and the world might seem scarier. We will all definitely meet death. I say let's use the inevitable as an opportunity to contribute and influence the top thinkers, designers, doers, carers, innovators, academics, policy-makers, change agents to make a difference to this sector – it is our time to shape not only what we want for our parents, but also for ourselves.

One project I have worked on in this area is *Alzheimers 100*, which I did as part of my role at Thinkpublic. We worked with Alzheimers Society, Dott07 and the Design Council to design ways to improve Dementia sufferers' daily lives in the North East, through the co-design of The Dementia Signposting Service. We worked closely with the regional community to understand what life was like for them, living with Dementia. To do this I created director's kits to capture the experiences of people with Dementia, and their carers' stories of living with someone with Dementia. We also designed and facilitated sessions in order to listen and meaningfully involve people in our co-design process, to understand where there were unmet needs and what sort of innovations would make a difference. This led to the design of a Dementia advisor role, which you can find out more about on the Alzheimers Society site (http://www.alzheimers.org.uk).

Even time can be designed for good use

As the creative director of *Spots of Time* I ran a pilot that aimed to encourage more volunteering in care homes across London and Essex. *Spots of Time* is a social enterprise with a mission to make it easier for people to put their spare 'spots of time' to good use in their communities. We created a range of fun, bite-sized activities for care homes to enable more volunteers to come into care homes, to improve the well-being of residents in our pilot across London and Essex. The pilot was a great example of rapid innovation – we worked with potential users – where we ran iterative testing phases to test what worked, and to learn and adapt the service in real time with users.

How to design your way out of a direct challenge or a barrier in five easy steps

1. *You do what?*
   I have found that care home managers aren't even sure of the more traditional roles of a designer, let alone the more innovative definition of a designer and how it might support them. Therefore, we must develop our skills as communicators to talk about the parts of our design brain that can support the challenges they may be facing.

2. *Work in partnership*
   We must leave our design egos at the door, and go in as facilitators and collaborators valuing absolutely everyone's value and contribution. We must work on our ability to facilitate and mediate so that we can bring out the expertise we see untapped, and not just rely on ourselves knowing the answers (because we don't).

3. *Demonstrate your capabilities*
   You may have to take on a small job like 'designing a logo' to demonstrate how you can add value. Demonstrating your capabilities goes miles further than being able to talk about your capabilities.

4. *Get buy in*

I have had most influence when I have been in positions where innovation projects have been well set up and organised, and with clear partnership at all levels. As a lone designer it is much harder; I have found myself spending loads of time working alongside organisations helping them to understand my contribution when it would have worked much better if my role had already been understood. When they 'get' what you do, it means they will potentially show a higher level of support.

5. *Don't do it alone*

I have also been able to offer more to organisations that are aligned with the vision I have set, by working collaboratively with other people and organisations. I do not have the single capacity/skills/influence as an individual.

There is a growing movement of designers who are putting their skills towards the contribution of the social good, and there are even more who are focussing on the challenges we face in the ageing sphere. We are on the right track; things are happening and there is more focus. If this is something you care about too, then I would encourage you to consider that now is probably a good time to join us – as in a few years we will already be on the wrong course. That is why we especially need designers to work together to shape the future of a thriving, ageing society.

Good luck!

Design for social innovation: the wisdom challenge

Virginia Tassinari

Social Spaces CUO, MAD Faculty (Belgium), DESIS Network

On a global scale, today's design community is witnessing an increasing number of social innovation projects, i.e. bottom up initiatives in which citizens collaboratively find new opportunities, and co-develop innovative solutions aimed at fulfilling societal needs. Examples include initiatives of community-supported agriculture (community gardens), co-housing, tool-sharing and so on. Each year the DESIS Network [1] – the international network of design for social innovation and sustainability – organises a series of events, in a variety of formats, often back-to-back with design events and Biennials.[A] One such format is the DESIS Showcase [3], during which we collect and present a kaleidoscope of cases of design for social innovation which are carried out from within an academic setting[B], Over the past two years, the Showcase event stands as a beautiful illustration of the exponential growth of case studies in social innovation. At the same time we have witnessed a growing interest in design-driven approaches to social innovation, from both public authorities and institutions and citizens in general.

The realities that most of these case studies represent exemplify a counter-trend to most mainstream developments and choices. They represent an acupuncture-like activation of the neuralgic points of communities and society, improving their resilience and abilities to heal and strengthen themselves, from within. Communities of people involved are enabled to look for and design solutions themselves, without always having to resort to a third party, e.g. welfare, institutions etc. The idea of a welfare state solving all societal issues for its citizens has been proven to be unsustainable, not only in economical terms but also in terms of the increasing complexity of society, which makes it difficult to apply one-size-fits-all, institutional top down measures. Hillary Cottam from the UK based collective, Participle, speaks about the

A See for instance, this year the Belgian Triennial of design Conflict and design www.conflictanddesign.be/

B Also in cooperation with Cumulus Association, http://www.cumulusassociation.org/

rise of 'relational welfare' [5], in which the collaborative bottom-up approach of social innovation-oriented initiatives is integrated with the top-down approaches of many, if not most, public and policy institutions. It is not either/or, but it is the complementarity between the two which is more likely to lead to a successful outcome. In the project 'The Circle Movement' [4], Cottam gives a practical example of the shape that relational welfare could take: i.e. to co-create a system with the elderly so that they can devise a common agenda where their activities, needs and resources are visualised. As such, they can basically help each other without needing to rely on social support structures. They can continue to live more independently in their own houses and steer their quality of life to a much larger extent.

Hence, welfare is supported by the same community, and something is attained which would have been impossible to reach otherwise, within the current economic and structural models. Empowered to help each other, the elderly rediscover the power of collaboration and the joy of being helpful to someone else. In this setting, the designer has taken on a role of enabling and empowering the elderly, of reading and translating their needs but also aspirations, and help them to act in order to make positive change happen. Rooted in a concrete local, real life context and working with real people with real needs and skills, one works to generate an internal resilience and a belief in continuity, so that as a designer one can slowly 'step back' from it. As such the project can grow and evolve beyond having to rely on the designer as the key engine of the system. It can become more than a mere design project to be featured in a magazine or shown at a conference, but rather, it can evolve into a working reality, with true societal impact. Once on its own legs, such projects can fuel a positive feedback-loop, which generates other unforeseen initiatives, hence becoming a catalyst of positive change.

With this approach, the designer aims to gain insight into people's needs and abilities and helps to bring them forward, not forgetting to design himself out of the system. Design for social innovation empowers the citizens by giving them the possibility to co-design and co-produce their own solutions. Ezio Manzini defines design for social innovation as "a constellation of design initiatives geared to making social innovation more probable, effective, long-lasting and apt to spread." [6]

The starting point is not a fixed idea in the designer's mind, but rather a given context with real people, real needs and real aspirations. In order to empower them to co-create their own solutions, one needs to explore new ways to create empathy and understand what is behind the untold, the personal stories, but also the story of the context, such as the symbolic value of places and objects. This requires a continuous search for the right instruments, since each case is different and requires different approaches. As such, the field of human and social sciences, as well as the fine and performing arts, represent an important sources of inspiration. They provide ingredients to further shape a sensitivity that can capture stories respecting their own uniqueness.

This goes for all stakeholders, yet especially when dealing with the elderly, there are many nuances at play. The past can be a key to reach the present, understand it and create a dialogue, even when it seems very complicated or even impossible, as in the case of Dementia. Alessia Cadamuro's project *What Remains?* is an example of how the entry point to a project can be represented by a reconstruction, through families and relatives, of stories that otherwise would have remained untold. What counts is not the seemingly insurmountable issue at stake – namely in this case the isolation of an elderly person affected by late-stage Dementia – but what can be read behind non-verbal cues that requirc special attention. Such cues can then be understood and translated into a tool that can empower the people involved and give them new opportunity to communicate and interact with each other. Beneath each issue lies an opportunity. The practice of design for social innovation points to a vast space of opportunity embodied by the elderly, as a valuable resource in our society, in need of further 'activation'. Our contemporary Western society appears to have un-learnt how to regard the elderly as having a specific authority and role within society. Developing countries and non-Western contemporary societies can remind us, or teach us, a lot in this respect, even if major changes are also taking place there.

It is not only an ethical issue to support the elderly in their everyday lives. We basically 'need' the elderly in order to really develop social innovation, as we need figures of reference, 'godfathers' that can be in charge of such initiatives, as they have both the time and the ability to do so, together with their desire to play a meaningful role. In order to guarantee the success of social innovation projects, we need a sense of continuity, dedicated people, who also have a historical memory of a place that can make sense of the state of the context in which a project is developed. Social innovation and the elderly are, as such, deeply inter-related, even when the projects have no specific focus on the elderly. Social innovation, in a way, is helping to re-think the role of the elderly as the wise, the pillars on which our society is built.

A further reflection is needed upon what this wisdom really entails, from an anthropological, sociological, ethnographical and philosophical perspective and to enrich the design discourse from the cultural perspective[C], If one looks at the origin of the word wisdom in ancient Greek, one encounters the idea of 'phronesis', which literally means the action to plan the best strategy possible in order to attain a better quality of life. It is surprising how close this definition comes to descibing the role that social innovation is aiming to give back to the elderly. Wisdom – i.e. this attitude to read beyond the mainstream to recognise what really matters in life, comes with time – and sometimes by having taken the wrong turn, and having learnt from these experiences. These are characteristics that I believe are also shared by design for social innovation. The latter takes time, requires patience and the ability to look at results in the long term, without focussing on the 'quick and easy'. There are many lessons to be learnt from wisdom as phronesis. Being wise does not necessarily mean to be too cautious, on the contrary: to be wise also means having the ability to recognise unexplored paths that can lead to something really valuable for one's own life, to be 'ingenuous', to look at the world through fresh, new eyes and to come up with surprising solutions. This does not mean that their potentiality is merely to have ideas and the resources to face issues related to the topic of ageing. Rather, they can help society to face all sorts of societal issues.

Over the past year, we have been working, together with Yanki Lee and Sara Hylten-Cavalliuson, on setting up the DESIS Cluster project entitled 'Ageing and Ingenuity' [2], an international cluster of projects of design institutions working on social innovation, which are inspired by the idea of seeing the elderly as an asset for the whole of society. We received tremendous response from all over the world, from China to Brazil, and from Japan to the US. The ability to work together on this issue with colleagues from so many countries will also allow us to identify cultural and sociological variables that play a role in design for social innovation within the context of the elderly, and offer us an opportunity to enrich each other's approaches in this way. Ageing is a well-recognised societal challenge, but I believe that what attracts so many schools to work on this issue is also a growing awareness that the elderly are not so much a societal problem to be solved, but instead they are a huge resource and opportunity for the whole of society. One could even go as far as to say that ideally, each project of design for social innovation should involve a mix of stakeholders from various age groups, including the elderly. On more than

C One possible platform for this discussion to take place is for instance the DESIS Philosophy Talks, series of discussions upon issues coming design for social innovation seen through philosophical lenses.

one occasion while working on such projects, we would declare that the input from the elderly was the pivotal factor in the project's success.

What we basically share in this context is the belief that a designer is well skilled to trigger the ingenuity of the elderly and their strong desire to be meaningful to their communities and societies. Through their wisdom they can help to ground more socially sustainable values and priorities, to co-design and co-produce new initiatives, which go in the direction of a more resilient and participatory society. Through this sharing of wisdom of the elderly in action, practitioners of design for social innovation can learn not only a lot themselves, but also help the elderly to rediscover the joy of being recognised as an indispensable foundation for our society. We strongly believe this to be a crucial challenge for social innovation, but also for (western) society at large. Hence collaboratively, we look forward to continuing on this path, undoubtedly paved with many insightful and rewarding surprises.

References

[1] *DESIS*. 2012. www.desis-network.org.

[2] Ageing Ingenuity, *DESIS*. 2012. www.desis-network.org/content/ageing-ingenuity.

[3] Showcase, *DESIS*. 2012. www.desis-showcase.org.

[4] The circle movement. *Participle*. 2013 www.participle.net/projects/view/5/101/.

[5] Cottam, H. *Relational Welfare*. Retrieved date? From Participle: www.participle.net/images/uploads/soundings48_cottam2.pdf.

[6] Manzini, E. (not dated) *Making things happen. Social innovation and design* Retrieved 30 September, 2013 from Social Innovation Generation: http://sigeneration.ca/documents/Makingthingshappen.pdf.

In a fast changing connected world, everybody designs. Professional designers, specifically, design experts, must help non-experts to design their lives. Therefore all design activities are, by definition, co-design activities. Ezio Manzini advocates design education institutions as important agents to drive this changing field. "It is not that designers have expanded their field of work to complex social situations, such as our ageing society, because they wanted to or felt like it. The issue is that the world is changed (this is not a rhetoric: it is true!). Therefore, the 'what' (and the 'how') of design have changed, too. Design experts today are simply trying to understand what they have to do, and how, in this new context. If design experts will or will not be able to have a positive role: that's another story... we are doing our best: aren't we?"

Design schools as agents of (sustainable) change

A Design Lab Network for an Open Design Programme

Ezio Manzini
DIS Politecnico di Milano – DESIS Network[A] first published: 18.05.2011

To educate someone to be a designer involves increasing his / her skills in conceiving and developing design proposals (from general visions to specific solutions) for a better world. The majority of these proposals can be seen as didactic exercises that usually end up in the teacher's archives and computer files. This generates an extensive amount of unused design work as well as a waste of students' and teachers' creativity, enthusiasm and expertise. In the past, this waste was, or was considered to be, inevitable. Today, in the transition towards fundamental and sustainable transformations on social, economic and environmental levels, facing the present demand for visions and solutions [12] and given the on-going changes in the design processes [11], this waste can be avoided: design school results and design student capabilities can become more socially effective and contribute to the solutions of the complex problems of contemporary society. How can it happen? To answer

A DESIS-Design for Social Innovation towards Sustainability is a network of design labs, based in design schools and design-oriented universities, actively involved in promoting and supporting sustainable change (www.desis-network.org).

this question we must consider the emerging scenario where open source [18] and peer-to-peer approaches [2] make possible new organisational framework and design networks: open and collaborative design processes where design schools can play an important role [6].

New scenario, new design

There is no doubt that today we are facing a deep (environmental, social, economic) crisis. At the same time, everybody agrees that the diffusion of networks and mobile technologies is opening new and, until now, unforeseeable possibilities. Finally, there is clearer and clearer evidence that these two mega-trends are converging and that, in doing so, they are generating new ideas and behaviours, new economies and, most importantly for us here, new design and production processes.

As a matter of fact, what this emerging scenario presents is a radical discontinuity with the models of the past century [13]. An exhaustive presentation is beyond the scope of this essay, but in order to discuss the possible role of design and design schools as agent of sustainable systemic change, two of its main features have to be outlined: the on-going shift from product to systems and services and from linear toward networked design processes.

Services and systems

In the emerging scenario, 'products' are complex entities, based on the interaction between people, products and places. For instance: distributed power generation systems (to optimise the use of diffuse and renewable energies); new food networks (to create direct links between cities and the countryside); intelligent mobility systems (to promote public transportation and innovative solutions); programmes of urban and regional development (to enhance local economies and new forms of community); collaborative services for prevention and healthcare (to involve directly interested users in the solution).

Considering these 'products' of the emerging scenario we can easily see that they are (mainly) technical and social networks, where people interact (and in turn interact with products and places) in order to obtain commonly recognised values. Operating in these networked systems, design (meant here as the design community of professional designers, design researchers, design academics and design media) shifts its focus from last century's product-oriented approach, towards a systemic one where the main attention is devoted to interactions. And where the 'objects' to be designed are a complex mix of material and immaterial systems of highly interconnected products, services, places and people [14] [8] [21] [7] [19].

New design networks

In the emerging scenario, designers (i.e. the experts who have been specifically trained in design-thinking and design-knowledge) are changing their position within production and consumption systems. In fact, the systemic changes they have to face are driven by a growing number of actors who together generate wide and flexible networks that collaboratively conceive, develop and manage sustainable solutions. Of course, in these new design networks the position and role of professional designers (the design experts) changes. Traditionally, designers have been seen and have seen themselves as the only creative members of interdisciplinary design processes. In the emerging scenario this clear distinction blurs, and they become professional designers among many non-professional ones. But even if this distinction blurs, it does not mean that the role of design experts is becoming less important. On the contrary, in this new context, design experts have the crucial function of bringing very specific design competences to these co-designing processes. That is, they become a particular kind of process facilitator, who uses specific design skills to enable the other actors to be good designers themselves [11] [12] [17] [5].

Thus design schools can play an important role in the emerging scenario and, more specifically, in these new design networks. They can generate original ideas and interact with local communities to trigger new initiatives or support the on-going ones.

Facilitating design networks

Design schools are, first and foremost, places where the next generation of design experts are educated. This fundamental educational role can be considered an investment on the future: if we want to build a better future, we have to prepare better people, in this case, better designers. However, to build a better future design schools now have the potential to play a second important role: that of agents of change: of critical and creative actors in the on-going transition towards sustainability, in a broader sense.

It is important to note that this second role (agents of change) largely reinforces the first one (to educate future generations of designers): as the world continues to undergo fundamental changes, the most effective way to prepare future (competent) designers is to involve students in problems, opportunities and design methods that today appear radically new and as yet involve only a small number of active minorities. Thanks to this involvement, students have the potential to play a meaningful role in contemporary society now (empowering the innovation processes that active minorities are generating), while simultaneously equipping themselves to be the leading designers of the future (when the problems, opportunities and design modalities that are emerging today will become the new standard). To this end, a design lab could be established within each school [6].

The expression 'Design Lab' refers to a team of researchers, teachers and students who orient their didactic and research activities towards promoting sustainable changes. As part of this process, they communicate with other similar labs, exchange experiences and join forces to give their results more visibility, and find potential partners with whom to build larger scenarios and solutions.

More precisely, what these design labs can do is to operate in peer-to-peer mode, as intelligent actors in new design networks. More precisely, they can use design classes and academic and professional design research to stimulate and support design networks in several ways:

- Investigating, exploring local resources and social innovation initiatives using ethnographic tools and user and community-centred design approaches to better understand problems and opportunities.
- Facilitating, supporting the co-design processes by using participative design tools to facilitate the interaction and convergence between the involved parties.
- Visioning, feeding the co-designing processes with scenarios and proposals at different scales: from the smallest (considering specific local problems), to the largest (aiming at building shared visions of the future).
- Communicating, giving the social innovation initiatives more visibility, explaining them and creating the pre-conditions to disseminate them, thanks to specifically designed communication programmes (websites, books, exhibitions, films, etc.).
- Enabling, empowering individuals and communities with dedicated solutions (the enabling solutions), which permit them to start and manage new and promising collaborative organisations.
- Replicating, scaling-up promising collaborative organisations and making

them more replicable, with the aid of toolkits and/or specifically conceived products and services.

- Synergising, promoting large-scale systemic changes and regional programmes by developing framework strategies, specifically conceived to both systemise and synergise a variety of local initiatives.

On-going projects

To better understand how design schools, via their design labs, can operate in the merging design networks, we can consider the concrete example of the Nutrire Milano project in Milano. Nutrire Milano (http://www.nutriremilano.it) is an on-going initiative aiming to regenerate the Milanese rural-urban agriculture (i.e. agriculture near the city) and at the same time offer organic and local food opportunities to the citizens by creating brand new networks of farmers and citizens based on direct relationships and mutual support.

This project is particularly meaningful in indicating what the role of a design lab could be. Years ago DIS (a didactic and research unit of the Indaco Department-Politecnico di Milano) started design classes and academic research on this theme. One year ago, in collaboration with the Slow Food Association and several other partners, it succeeded in promoting the Nutrire Milano project, founded by a bank foundation (the Fondazione Cariplo), to be implemented over the following five years [15]. In this example, the design classes had the role of preparing the ground for implementation of the project. First of all, they facilitated the recognition of existing (social, cultural and economic) local resources and best practices. Moving from here, they outlined a strategy, considering the emerging trends towards a new possible synergy between cities and the countryside (similar to those towards zero-mile food and proximity tourism). Finally, on this basis, they built a shared and socially recognised vision: the vision of a rural-urban area where agriculture flourishes while feeding the city, and at the same time offers citizens opportunities for a multiplicity of farming and nature-related activities [16].

Now, the project has moved on from the design class and academic research stage and is ready for implementation. It is remarkable that, thanks to this preliminary work, a large project like this (planned to last five years and involving a very wide regional area) has already obtained its first concrete result (the huge success of the farmers market) in less than one year since starting up. We should add that two new initiatives will be started in the next two years and that several others are programmed for implementation in the future.

Other initiatives similar to the Nutrire Milano project can be found worldwide: in several design schools teams of researchers, teachers and students are working on projects that increasingly involve other outside players and generate social consensus, political will and economic resources to become real world, operative programmes. Just to quote two well-known cases, we can point to the Chongming Eco-community project, in Shanghai (http://chongmingtao.blogspot.com) and the Amplify Project, in New York (http://desis.parsons.edu). But, to be sure, the list of cases will continue and expand in all regions of the world (for more examples, see www.desis-network.org and www.sustainable-everyday.net).

In conclusion of this part, we can say that these examples give clear indications of what the role of design school lab has been and could be, in promoting sustainable changes, mixing didactic and research activities in schools and collaborating with various stakeholders in real world projects. We can observe that design labs start, develop and coordinate this kind of project in different ways and at different scales: from local (where they co-design specific initiatives with local actors) to regional (where they cooperate with other stakeholders in the definition and implementation of large framework projects). To do that, specific strategic design capabilities are needed to recognise the existing resources and best practices, evaluate on-going influential trends, involve the stakeholders and facilitate their convergence toward shared visions, and common decisions on what to do and how. In parallel, when local projects start to take shape, design experts must collaborate in synergising them and coordinating them with other on-going and/or future programmes. Finally, and most importantly, the overall project and each one of the local ones must be effectively communicated to those involved (and potentially involved) and towards a larger audience, which must be made aware of what the overall project is doing, and what it will do, step by step [10] [9].

Open Design Programme[B]

The previous examples are significant because they demonstrate how some schools have become agents of (sustainable) change. At the same time, they show the possibilities connected to this way of working and the potential implicit in a diffused network of similar labs in several design schools. To advance such an approach calls for the development of a far-reaching design and research programme [12].

B Not to be confused with the Open Design Spaces at Design Academy Eindhoven, which are referred to throughout the publication [ed.].

To be effective, such a programme should be unique in its concept and realisation: a design programme based on a peer-to-peer approach, including design schools from all over the world. The programme should be both open and collaborative, and capable of self-regulation and self-management. We can name it Open Design Programme.

The expression Open Design Programme refers to a programme of (didactic and research) initiatives where several design teams are challenged by significant and complex problems and collaborate to produce shared visions and viable solutions. This requires an appropriate communication and organisation platform. It must enable the design lab to operate adopting open source and peer-to-peer approaches to exchange experiences, mutually evaluate their projects and, finally, collaborate in large programmes.

The Open Design Programme we are proposing here is characterised by these features and has three primary goals: (1) to define a shared framework for a multiplicity of research activities on design and sustainability; (2) to create a forum for on-going discussion and outline design and research streams on well defined crucial issues and emerging scenarios; (3) to foster new autonomous research programmes.

The design labs that join this programme agree to orient their on-going activities, or start new ones, in such a way that they can tackle these crucial issues and enrich these emerging scenarios. In doing this, these labs offer their contribution to the realisation of an articulated set of visions and proposals (as well as the definition of design tools necessary to better understand and implement them). At the same time, the programme operates as a platform enabling each design lab to recognise emerging demands, exchange experiences with those working on similar topics, and have greater access to design tools and concepts developed and tested in other projects.

Distributed Design Agency

To enhance the Open Design Programme, each design lab develops projects and research on the basis of its own resources and opportunities, but also acts as a node within a larger network of similar labs. What results is a Design Lab Network which operates as an innovative design agency: both as an open agency [17], where complex, socially significant topics can be tackled, scenarios developed, and solutions offered as contributions to larger innovation and co-design processes; and as a distributed agency [4], where many design teams

work in parallel, are connected to each other and can function as a larger entity, while remaining sensitive to particular local cultural, social, and economic conditions. Given its particular system architecture this design lab network offers the very unique possibility to integrate local and global points of view and to promote open design programmes where a variety of projects converge, untangling complex problems and generating scenarios and solutions.
In other words, the Design Lab Network is, per se, a kind of social innovation where, as we wrote at the beginning, the existing (but under-valued) social resource of students' enthusiasm and teachers' experience is catalysed and realised to generate a distributed design agency where scenarios and solutions, conceptual frameworks and practical tools are generated and offered as a free and open contribution to the on-going co-designing processes towards sustainability.

It must also be emphasised that this distributed design agency is primarily and most importantly an independent design agency: one based in design schools and which can operate with greater degrees of freedom than commercial design agencies. We believe that the freedom to search for unconventional, critical, alternatives is the major strength of the Design Lab Network and Open Design Programme.

In acting as independent agents of change, design schools are doing precisely what they should do: operate as free cultural entities capable of using that freedom to promote social good, even when this contradicts mainstream models.

References

[1] Bauwens, M. 2006. *The Political Economy of Peer Production in Post-autistic economics review*. Retrieved date 5 October 2013 from http://www.ctheory.net/articles.aspx?id=499.

[2] Bauwens, M. 2007. Peer to Peer and Human Evolution, *Foundation for P2P Alternatives*, p2pfoundation.net.

[3] Biggs C, Ryan C, Wiseman J, Larsen K. *Distributed Water Systems: A networked and localised approach for sustainable water services*. Victorian Eco Innovation Lab, Melbourne, 2009.

[4] Biggs, C., Ryan, C. Wisman, J. Distributed Systems. *A design model for sustainable and resilient infrastructure, VEIL Distributed Systems BriefingPaper N3*, University of Melbourne, Melbourne, 2010.

[5] Brown, T., Wyatt, J. Design Thinking for Social Innovation, *Stanford Social Innovation review*, Winter, 2010.

[6] *DESIS*, 2009, http://www.desis-network.org.

[7] Green, J, *Democratizing the future: towards a new era of creativity and growth*. Koninklijke Philips Electronics N.V, Eindhoven, 2007.

[8] Halen, C., Vezzoli, C., & Wimmer, R. *Methodology for product service system innovation*. Uitgeverij Koninklijke Van Gorcum, Assen, 2005.

[9] Jégou, F. Social innovations and regional acupuncture towards sustainability, *Zhuangshi*. China ZHUANGSHI Journal Agency, Beijing, 2010.

[10] Jégou, F. Manzini, E., *Collaborative services Social Innovation and design for sustainability*. Poli.Design, Milan, 2008.

[11] Leadbeater, C. *We-Think*. Profile Books, London, 2008.

[12] Manzini, E. New Design Knowledge, in *Changing the Change*, Design Studies, 2009.

[13] Manzini, E. Small, Local, Open and Connected: Design Research Topics in the Age of Networks and Sustainability, in *Journal of Design Strategies*, Volume 4, No. 1, Spring, 2010.

[14] Manzini, E., Collina, L, Evans, S, (Eds.), *Solution oriented partnership. How to design industrialised sustainable solutions*, UK, 2004.

[15] Meroni, A. Strategic Design to take care of the territory. Networking Creative Communities to link people and places in a scenario of sustainable development, in *P&D Design São Paulo*, Brazil, 2008.

[16] Meroni, A., Simeone, G. Trapani, P. Envisioning sustainable urban countryside: Service Design as contribute to the rururban planning in *Cumulus Working Papers – St. Etienne*, edited by Justyna Maciak, Camille Vilain and Josyane Franc, University of Art and Design Helsinki. 2009.

[17] Mulgan, G. Steinberg, T. Salem, O. *Wide Open: Open source methods and their future potential*, Demos Publications, 2005.

[18] Murray, R., Caulier-Grice, J., Mulgan, G. *The Open Book of Social Innovation*. NESTA Innovating Public Services, London, 2010.

[19] Pauli, G. *The Blue Economy*. Paradigm Publications, US, 2010.

[20] *SEP*, 2010, http://www.sustainable-everyday.net.

[21] Thackara, J. *In the bubble, Designing in a complex world*, The MIT Press, London, 2005.

[22] Verganti, R. *Design-Driven Innovation*, Harvard Business press, 2009.

[23] von Hippel, E. *The Democratization of Innovation*. MIT Press, Cambridge, MA, 2004.

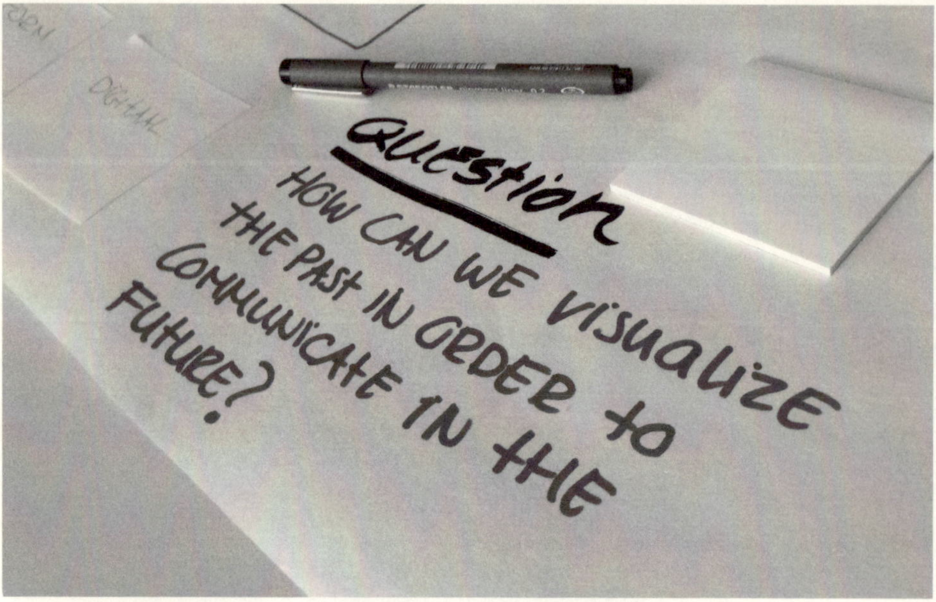

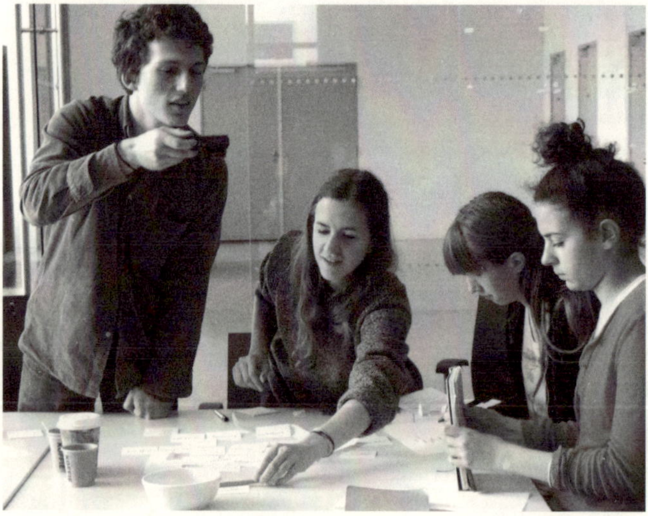

What Remains?
Open Design Space,
work session.

Open Design Space
Designing with empathy

Jacqueline Cové

The Open Design Space (ODS) *What Remains?* at Design Academy Eindhoven focussed on patients with late-stage Dementia, which, in view of the ageing global population, is a very topical and socially relevant subject. Two questions played a central role in the short course: "How can a more empathic design approach create a better understanding between carers and patients?" and, "Can we create tools to improve communication with patients of Alzheimer's disease?" Working with new design research methods and skills, such as empathic design, thinking-through-discussion and thinking-through-making approach, students were given the opportunity to find new ways to acquire knowledge and come up with ideas. As a teacher at Design Academy Eindhoven I was asked to participate in the ODS as tutor. In this text I will explain what these design methods and skills meant for the ODS, and what they could mean for design education at large.

1. Empathic design approach

The ODS *What Remains?* was initiated by Alessia Cadamuro. She gave a description of the Dementia disease to the students and set assignments based on an empathic research method. Students had to identify with a carer or imagine the world for a person with Dementia.[1] During these conversations students questioned their own ideas by listening to those of others. Visualising the outcomes (emotions) with a mind map resulted in a list of keywords for further research. This helped students to immerse into the world of the patient and the carer. As Daniël van Ginkel reflected: "The empathic research was surprisingly effective. Taking time to imagine what it would mean to be a patient or carer really worked... Eventually this mental immersing resulted in a collective understanding of what we think is the situation of people dealing with Dementia. Of course this is solely based on our own experiences and is relatively subjective. Nevertheless I did get the feeling we were close to a realistic point of view and understanding." The students used their imagination, intuition, sensitivity and empathy as design skills and became more aware of the patients' state of mind. The process of exchanging experiences and reusing ideas created new ones. As students emphasised during the meetings

– the strength of an empathic research approach is applicable to many more areas than just dealing with patients with Dementia.

2. Sharing / Outsider – Insider

Students were given the opportunity to talk to a professional carer from Careyn, an aged care facility, and patients' relatives in the role of carers (referred to in Dutch as 'mantelzorgers'). The carer gave more information about working with Dementia patients in general, in care homes, such as a lack of personal information about patients. The relatives gave a more personal and emotional account. These conversations produced a lot of information and stimulated the process. Students came to a better understanding of the complexity of Dementia. The discussion helped them focus on personal questions and ideas. As student Alexander Marinus wrote: "The carer spoke about the creative therapist who would paint and sculpt with the patients, and the reactions this caused in some of the patients, which triggered me to formulate my research question: What is the relationship between 'creating' and our memory?"

3. Connecting / Co Design

Valentijn Visch (TU Delft, project leader of the CRISP G-Motiv project, p. 35) and Tom Bieling from Design Research Lab in Berlin2 both emphasised the importance of multidisciplinary teams and stressed that designers should concern themselves with societal issues. For many students this was a key reason to participate in the ODS. Students feel the urge to work on real issues that society faces. Projects such as *What Remains?* gave them a taste of the role design can play as they became acquainted with methods to work on issues concerning healthcare.

From an educational standpoint it is important that students meet professionals from other fields. Tom Bieling's visit proved to be an eye-opener, since his design practice mainly deals with problems of communication, and is often a result of co-designing and sometimes the result of community-based ideas.

4. From design research to design research proposals

During the design research process the question 'Can we create tools to improve communication with patients of Alzheimer's disease?' resulted in different personal research questions from the students. The questions concentrated on three main subjects: the role of our memories, communication opportunities using our senses, and storing personal information. During the last meeting the students were asked to explain their process to Bas Raijmakers (Reader in Strategic Creativity at DAE, see his text on p. 69) and Alice Osborne (Design and Communications at My HomeLife, London, find her text on p. 41). Some of the results were text-based, analysing a problem with a clear proposal at the end, such as Sandra Lundberg's proposal for 'a sensory library that can stimulate memory and encourage expression (verbal or non-verbal)'. Others presented a visualisation of thoughts, words and pictures giving an impression of the design research area. Laura Koenen presented a 'memory book' of her mother and Tom van 't Westeinde elaborated on a Dementia project running at the TU/e. This exchange and sharing between the students and guests was inspiring. Sandra Lundberg stated: "It lead to conclusions I would have never reached on my own. I don't believe in the lonely designer; I believe in working together."

Allow me to digress briefly. The ratio of students / tutors was 11: 2, providing this ODS the luxury position of having invited a great number of professionals with such varied backgrounds and that they all excepted. The mix of students (students from various levels, a master student, a TU/e student and an Artez Zwolle student) enriched the quality of the reflections and discussions. Though the students could have been a little bit more critical towards each other (they were very kind and understanding – maybe a little too empathic), and would as such gain more from the weekly meetings and progress more with their projects.

All in all, the ODS *What Remains?* was a success: the students (who participated on a voluntary basis) were highly motivated and enthusiastic. The variety of guests was incredibly valuable. It gave students the opportunity to acquire new design research skills that can be applied to any other design context. In my opinion, design education could benefit from including these methods in the regular educational programme. Students would acquire an exciting and innovative design research attitude, an asset in the constantly changing design field.

References

[1] B. Raijmakers, G. van Dijk, Y. Lee and S. A. Williams, Designing Empathic Conversations for Inclusive Design Facilitation, presented at Include09, Royal College of Art, London, UK, 5-8 April 2009.
[2] Information on his contribution to the Mobile Lorm Glove, which enables deaf-blind people to communicate, can be found here: http://www.design-research-lab.org/?projects=mobile-lorm-glove, accessed 5 October 2013.

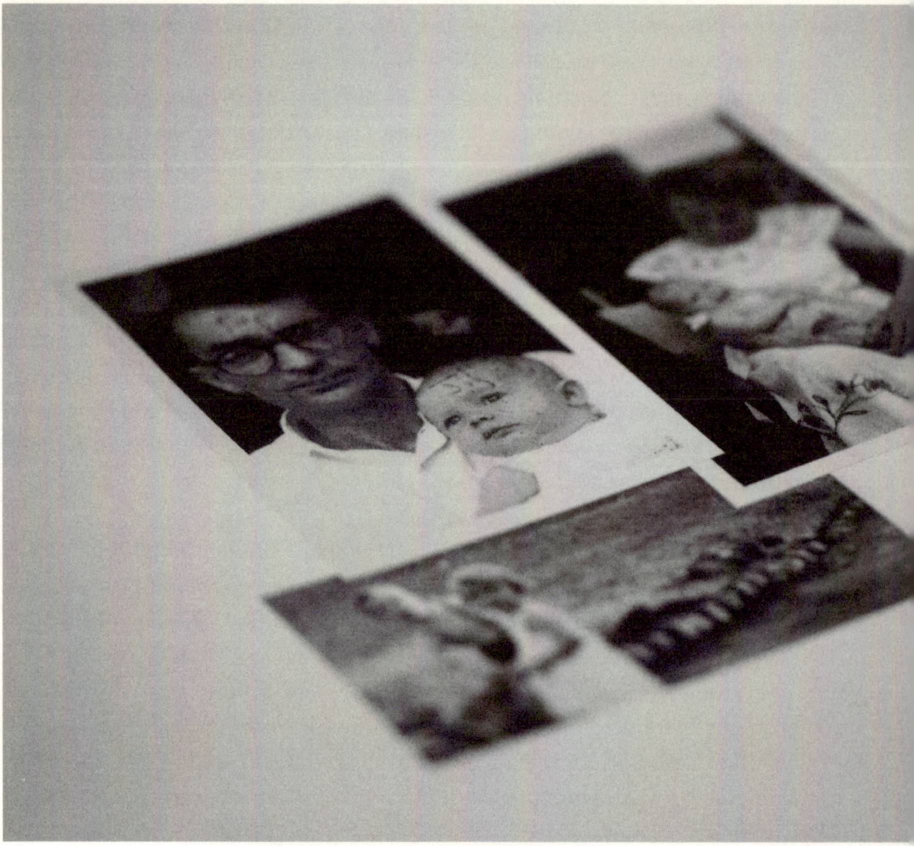

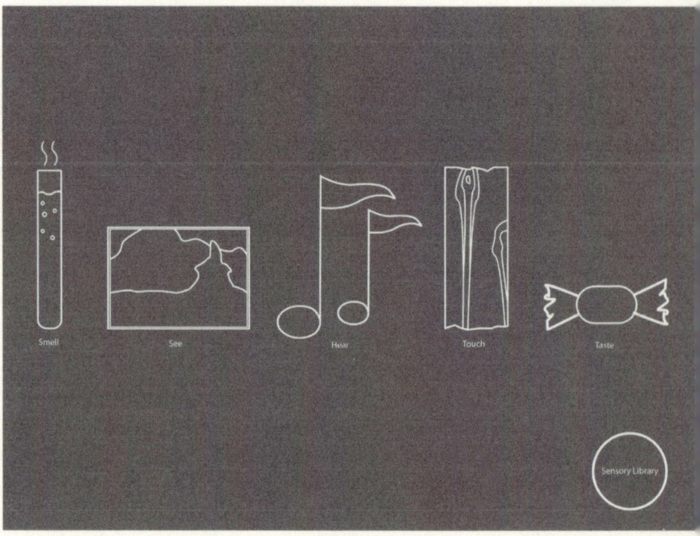

Sandra Lundberg, Design Academy student presented a multisensory stimulation project to facilitate storytelling to elderly patients with Dementia.

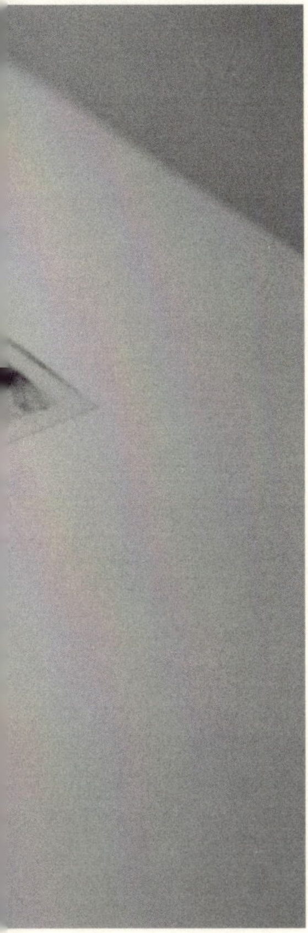

Laura Koenen, Design Academy student designed a written and photographic diary to be used in special scenarios and before the eventual diagnosis of Dementia. Her mother has a high chances of acquiring Dementia in the future for genetic reasons, therefore she is already preparing for this eventuality by creating her personal memory diary.

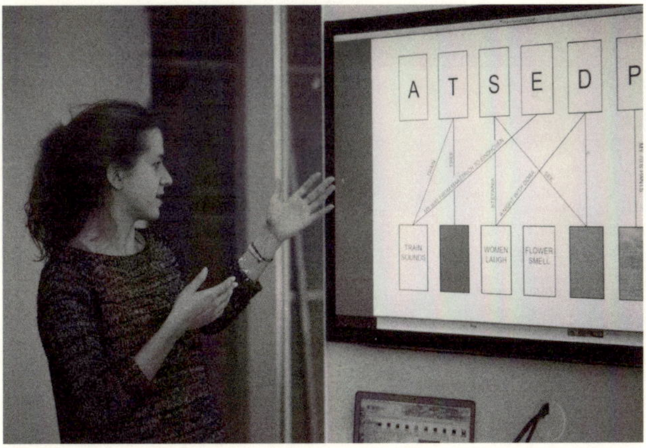

Clémence Althabegoïty, Design Academy student designed as a result of *What Remains?* ODS a card game that can help elderly with Dementia to stimulate logic connections through memories.

The contribution of *What Remains?* to CRISP

Bas Raijmakers

What Remains? is part of one of the eight main projects within the CRISP programme called G-Motiv - Changing Human Behaviour Using Game-Elements, and its results move the overall goals of CRISP ever forward. CRISP is a four-year project, which started in 2011 and will end in 2015, with many connected, small projects within it. Through these project contributions, CRISP also becomes more concrete, as a vehicle to make design more strategic and render society more resilient, through design.

The power of Product Service Systems: design and deliver on several levels simultaneously

CRISP focuses on Product Service Systems (PSS) because holistic approaches that simultaneously look at products, systems and services work best when dealing with many of the complex problems our society is facing. Problems immune to simple or quick fixes require an approach that embraces complexity, by trying to understand the situation rather than simplify it. The growing number of people with Dementia is one such complex situation. First and foremost, Dementia affects patients and their families and friends on an extremely personal level. But also on societal, cultural and even global levels Dementia has its effects, for instance on rising health care costs, or at an ethical level when we have to consider what sort of care is still humane. *What Remains?* enters this area with the kind of confidence that comes from a design approach that is firmly grounded in the daily lives and practices of the people involved. On the personal level, *What Remains?* made meaningful changes to the lives of the patients and their carers, who took part in the design research and used the prototype. The professional carers noted how a deeper understanding of their patients could ease the care work they do every day. It also made their work more meaningful because since participating in the project they have been able to get to know their patients better, and are more equipped to cater for their (mental) needs. These personal benefits eventually have their effect on societal and cultural levels, obviously when the care becomes more humane and easier to deliver.

Designers have a strategic role to play in making society more resilient

Starting from a deep empathy with the people with Dementia and their carers (professionals and family) Alessia Cadamuro wrote her own brief, working on many levels, as researcher, product designer, service designer and game designer. Always taking a holistic approach in her design research, this resulted in a true Product Service System: the service she created centres around care for people with late-stage Dementia, in care homes. The system consists of the collection, organisation and use of photos and notes related to the previous life of the patient. The product is a number of spherical objects to play a photo game between patient and informal carer. The collaboration between professional carer and family or friends of the patient, often informal carers, links all this together, which makes *What Remains?* so special. Together they form a team: the informal carer searching for photos and stories from the family to play the game, and professional carers using the understanding gathered about the patients to deliver more bespoke care. Coincidentally, seriously growing collaboration between informal and professional carers is one of the very few existing visions that would allow to maintain the current quality of care in the face of growing demand and dwindling resources. *What Remains?* brings that vision to fruition in a very elegant way. Such PSSs are not simply commissioned in a design brief by an organisation. They emerge rather, from deep, empathic design research by designers who are not scared away by initial failures and institutional hurdles. These designers basically write their own briefs in collaboration with the people who live through these situations every day. Writing your own brief in such a way is fundamentally strategic of course, because it grows out of cumulative insights that allow designers to take new, grounded directions.

How can design education prepare designers for such roles?

Design Academy Eindhoven students quickly realised that the care for people with late-stage Dementia is very complex when they got the opportunity to talk to professional and informal carers in the Open Design Space organised by Alessia Cadamuro and Jacqueline Cové. Visits from designers working with patients with Dementia offered a chance to see how designers have found meaningful ways to intervene and contribute in this area. However, the many expertises, skills and perspectives needed to address such problems are often difficult to bring to life in education, simply because bringing many people (experts, carers and designers dealing with Dementia, for instance) into a class is cost prohibitive and takes a great deal of effort to organise on a weekly basis.

Yet, as Jacqueline Covée observes in her text, the variety of guests in the Open Design Space was incredibly valuable because the students acquired essential design research skills they can use in any design project. So how to make this approach affordable? Creating a connection between education and academic design research offers a solution. Design researchers create a network of experts and collaborators around them over time, and can offer this network to education. This becomes financially viable as well when educational and research planning are flexible enough (or are designed to be!) to make visits of people from this network doubly beneficial: for the design researcher and students.

Alessia Cadamuro has been pioneering such double benefits with her design of the Open Design Space *What Remains?* together with DAE tutor Jacqueline Covée. It is fair to say that this kind of education design moves beyond mere teaching. Rather, the Open Design Space was curated from a deep understanding of how design has contributed to Dementia care over the past decade, and from a service design perspective that is empathetically involved in Dementia care, including its patients. This demonstrates that CRISP contributes to new approaches in design education on a strategic level, by creating and exploring new bridges between design education and academic design research.

Contributor biographies

Daniëlle Arets

Associate Reader (Associate Lector) in the Readership (Lectoraat) Strategic Creativity, Daniëlle Arets also possesses a key role in communicating the knowledge that results from CRISP to creative industries and education as a Knowledge Transfer Officer for CRISP. Arets has a strong record in organising debates for a wide array of public, educational and commercial institutes, and through this experience she has become a strong advocate for interdisciplinary research and design. As Associate Lector and Knowledge Transfer Officer, Danielle aims to bridge academic and design thinking through strategic, creative tools and techniques, and of course, many debates.

Alessia Cadamuro

Alessia Cadamuro is a researcher and designer who brings a strong sense of empathy and humanity in her work to co-create solutions focussing on real people with real histories. She has a multidisciplinary approach to design because she strongly believes in the deep value of the collaboration between different disciplines and specialisations. Her work touches relevant design and social issues, such as the role which design could play in humanising service systems in relation to sensitive areas, and to the new possibilities that this could create in a future society. Cadamuro completed her Bachelor of Architecture at the University of Iuav in Venice, Italy, and consequently obtained her MDes at the Man and Humanity department at Design Academy Eindhoven, The Netherlands. As part of CRISP she is as Research Associate at Design Academy Eindhoven involved in the G-Motiv project.

Jacqueline Covë

Jacqueline Covë has been teaching Art History since 1985 when she started working at Hogeschool voor de Kunsten, Artez. Following this, she also accepted a position at Design Academy Eindhoven, where her focus lies on design history. Over the years she has been involved in various projects that deal with research, debate, reflection and theory and she has expanded her teaching to the fields of graphic, animation and comic design. In 2012 she was one of the co-founders of a new platform for debate in Utrecht, House of Commons.

Ré Dubhthaigh

Ré Dubhthaigh is a founder and principal of The Civic Works, Ireland, where he leads on service strategy work with public sector organisations including Dublin City Council, the Department of Health and the Crafts Council of Ireland. He has a background in design research and strategy. As director of service design agency, Radarstation, he has led projects for clients including BBC, Sony, Lego, Southern Water, and Hitachi. Dubhthaigh is a Design Associate at the UK Design Council, working with start-ups and industry and public sector organisations in the UK to innovate their services. Dubhthaigh has an MA in Interaction Design from the Royal College of Art, London, and has been a researcher at InnovationRCA and the Interaction Design Institute, Ivrea. He is a regular lecturer and speaker on design and service strategy internationally, and was an advisory panel member for Pivot, Dublin's World Design Capital bid in 2010.

Bas Raijmakers

Dr. Bas Raijmakers PhD (RCA) is Reader (Lector) in Strategic Creativity at Design Academy Eindhoven and leads the in-house CRISP research team. Bas Raijmakers has a background in cultural studies, the internet industry, and interaction design. His main passion is to bring the people for whom we design into design and innovation processes, using visual storytelling. He holds a PhD in Design Interactions from the Royal College of Art, in London. He is also co-founder and Creative Director of STBY in London and Amsterdam: a design research consultancy specialised in design research for service innovation. Bas Raijmakers works for clients in the public sector and industry, around the globe.

Ezio Manzini

For more than two decades Ezio Manzini has been working in the field of design for sustainability. Recently, he has focussed his interests on social innovation, and established and coordinates, DESIS: an international network on design for social innovation and sustainability (http://www.desis-network.org). Throughout his professional life he worked at the Politecnico di Milano, where now he is Honorary Professor. Parallel to this, he collaborated with several international schools, such as the Domus Academy (in the 90s), Hong Kong Polytechnic University (in 2000) and, currently, Tongji University (Shanghai), Jiangnan University (Wuxi), COPPE-UFRJ (Rio de Janeiro) and Parsons (New York).

Alice Osborne

Alice Osborne is a designer with a diverse range of skills in health and social care, aging, and end of life. She works on projects where she can give away all she knows to forward thinking and innovative people, projects and organisations in their approach to helping us live well as we age, and prepare and face the end of our lives. She was a speaker at the ODS What Remains? at Design Academy Eindhoven and mentored some of the projects on the way that they were using design to approach innovative ideas around aging. If you'd like to follow her journey, you can do so here @AliceOsborne.

Virginia Tassinari

After her studies in philosophy Virginia Tassinari became interested in connecting the world of philosophy and design. She applies the study of criticism of society to the contemporary context, which she translates to the design world with design projects that work on the border between of philosophy and society. Actively engaged in teaching at the Media, Arts and Design (MAD) Faculty Belgium she develops socially relevant projects and collaborates with different initiatives in the field of social innovation and its relationship with philosophy. She is guest lecturer at different universities, such as George Brown University Toronto and Politecnico di Milano. Recently she founded a DESIS Lab within her research group Social Spaces in MAD Faculty. Furthermore she feeds the discourse with the initiative of the DESIS Philosophy Talks, which she initiated with Prof. Ezio Manzini and Prof. Victor Margolin as well as through her function of board member of Cumulus, the international Association of Universities of Art, Media and Design.

Valentijn Visch

Valentijn Visch (1971) works as assistant professor at the faculty of Industrial Design at the Delft University of Technology. He conducts and coordinates persuasive game design research, and is project leader of the Economic Affairs funded CRISP G-Motiv project (2011-2015) and the NWO granted NextLevel project (2013-2017). Both research projects contain research, industry and user-organizational partners. Visch has a background in Literature (MA), Art theory (MA – postgraduate Jan van Eijck Academy), Animation (postgraduate NIAF Tilburg), Cultural Sciences and film studies (PhD – VU), and experimental emotion research.

Colophon

What Remains?

The Readership in Strategic Creativity at Design Academy Eindhoven

Editor:	Alessia Cadamuro
Editorial team:	Daniëlle Arets, Ré Dubhthaigh, Bas Raijmakers, Ellen Zoete
Writers:	James M. Boekbinder, Jacqueline Cové, Ré Dubhthaigh, Alice Osborne, Bas Raijmakers, Virginia Tassinari, Valentijn Visch
Proofreader:	Jane Hardjono
Graphic design:	Eric de Haas
Printed by:	Lecturis, Eindhoven
Edition:	500

CRISP research group:

G-Motiv

CRISP partners:

Delft University of Technology, Careyn, Monobanda

Guest tutor Open Design Space:

Jacqueline Cové

Participating students Open Design Space:

Daniël Gaciu, Daniël van Ginkel, Archibald Godts, Laura Koenen, Laura van der Kruijs, Sandra Lundberg, Cecilia Maarawi, Alexander Marinus, Egle Ugintaite, Clemence Althabegoity, Tom van 't Westeinde.

Special thanks to:

Swanny Meijdam-Blokzijl, Tonko Blokzijl and Marja Dijkwel, Zhenya Pashkina and Monobanda

Publisher:
Design Academy Eindhoven
Emmasingel 14
Eindhoven, The Netherlands
www.designacademyeindhoven.nl/strategiccreativity
email: opendesignspaces@designacademy.nl

ISBN: 978-94-91400-11-7
Price: 10 euro

The Readership in Strategic Creativity, 2013
Reader (Lector): Dr Bas Raijmakers PhD (RCA)
Associate Reader (Associate Lector): Drs Daniëlle Arets
Visiting Research Fellow: Ré Dubhthaigh MA (RCA)
Research Associates: Michelle Baggerman BA, Alessia Cadamuro MDes, Heather Daam MDes, Maartje van Gestel BA, Susana Cámara Leret MDes, Karianne Rygh MDes, Mike Thompson MDes, Jonathan Wray MDes

The Readership Strategic Creativity is partly funded within the Creative Industry Scientific Programme (CRISP). CRISP is supported by the Dutch Ministry of Education, Culture and Science. www.crispplatform.nl

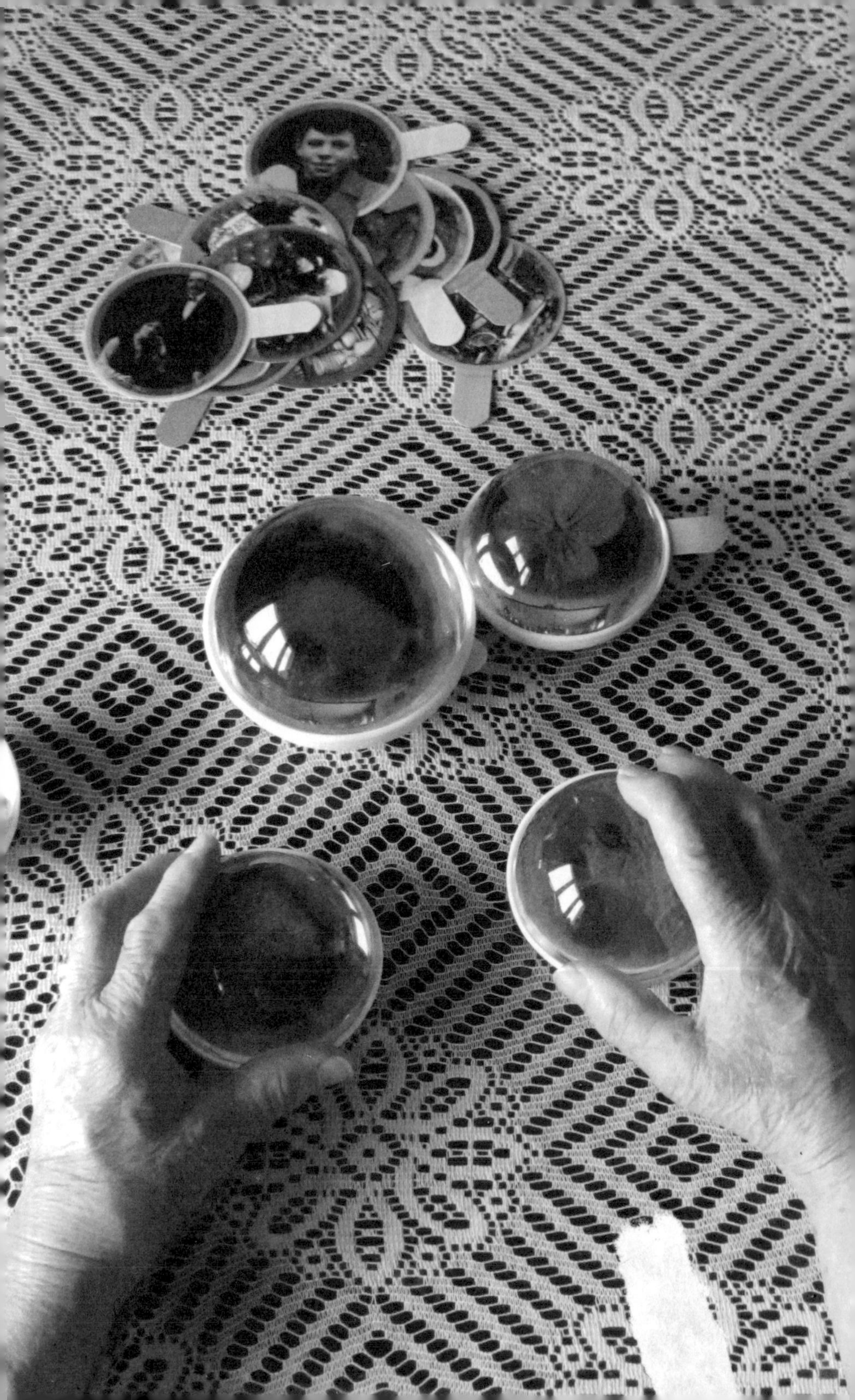